中醫簡學

Traditional Chinese Medicine Simplified

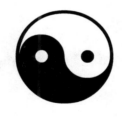

By

Ko Tan

ISBN 0-7414-2936-5

Illustrations and Digital Graphics by: Ko Tan, Terry Palmer, and Dover Publications, Inc.

Text Design and Layout by: Ko Tan

Cover Art by: Cheng, Tung Heng

Cover Design by: Ko Tan and Infinity Publishing Company

Published by:

INFINITY
PUBLISHING.COM

1094 New DeHaven Street, Suite 100
West Conshohocken, PA 19428-2713
Info@buybooksontheweb.com
www.buybooksontheweb.com
Toll-free (877) BUY BOOK
Local Phone (610) 941-9999
Fax (610) 941-9959

Printed in the United States of America
Printed on Recycled Paper
Published April 2006

Dedicated to the memory of
my parents, who were always my supporters in life and
who inspired me to achieve all that life has to offer.
Thank you for your love.

****

Acknowledgments

All my teachers of past, present, and future: Thank you for your teachings, wisdom, knowledge, and love.

Christine Issel: Without you this book would never have come into existence. I thank you for all the time and effort you put into editing the manual that later became this book. Thanks for questioning all the not-so-clear ideas and helping me to express them in words. Most of all, thanks for caring.

Carole Addlestone: Thanks for spending your valuable time proofreading the drafts before the printing of this book.

David Dunn, Thomas Branch, and Josh Lane: Thanks for your wonderful help, information, and friendships.

Dr. Bruce Costello: Thank you for offering Rising Spirit Institute as a launching pad for this more-than-eight-years' project.

Terry Palmer: Thank you for the digital graphics. They look great.

My clients, my students, friends, and others who have come into my life: Thanks for cheering me on through the writing of this book.

Bryan K. Busby (Keithie): Thank you for being in my life and for giving me the whole-hearted support, care, and love I needed most.

Traditional Chinese Medicine Simplified

Contents

Part I: History & Theory

Part II: Practical Application of TCM

Introduction

My students are mostly Westerners. *Traditional Chinese Medicine Simplified* came out of my need to introduce a different language, concepts of thinking, and the culture of Traditional Chinese Medicine (TCM) to these students. The search for information led me to explore a number of available texts. I found that most are truly insightful although more in depth than needed for the beginning-level student. My hope is not to undermine the vast concepts and thoughts behind the age-old wisdom and knowledge but to simplify TCM in order to help many come to a basic level of understanding on this complex subject. I am indebted to all the authors and writers who have paved the way for me to create this book. In addition, I thank all my teachers who have taught me many forms of bodywork as well as self-help exercises.

While teaching, I found that my students needed more than just theory to have a deeper grasp of the subject. I began to add the applications of TCM in my classes. The students' understanding of the subject jumped to a new height after learning how to utilize this foreign concept in their daily lives. Part II of this book applies the concepts of Part I.

The more I wrote, the more I wanted to include in each chapter. I wanted to put more explanations, more illustrations, and more topics. Finally I had to put a stop to it, saying to myself that to include more is to undo the simplification I was striving for. I backed off from all the emotional attachments and went ahead and produced this textbook. My apology to anyone who finds that this book strips away the essence of the wisdom of TCM. That is not my intention.

It is my wish that this book be of great help to many in understanding and applying the concepts of TCM, and that teachers find it an easy text from which to instruct. Please note, however, that the Yin and Yang Organs in TCM are not the actual physical forms as understood in Western thinking.

I encourage everyone to use my bibliography at the end of this book as a resource to explore further the depth and richness of TCM.

Love and peace,
Ko Tan

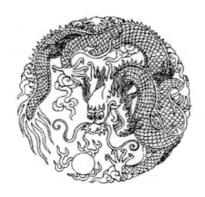

Part 1:
History & Theory

歷
史
及
理
論

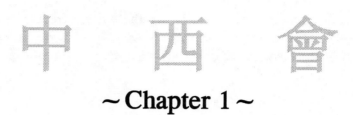

~ Chapter 1 ~

East Meets West: Expanding One's Viewpoint

"It is possible there exists human emanations that are still unknown to us. Do you remember how electrical currents and 'unseen waves' were laughed at? The knowledge about man is still in its infancy."
—Albert Einstein

"Energy cannot be seen and understood except through its material manifestations."
—Chinese Classic Nei Ching Ling Shu, two thousand years ago

Quantum Physics

Quantum physics is the branch of physics that studies the energetic characteristics of matter at the sub-atomic level. It deals not so much with material things, but with fields of energy, with this dynamic force within objects. Pioneers in the quantum physics field include Albert Einstein, Max Plank, and Neils Bohr. They developed the work that uncovered the dual nature of electrons. Electrons behave both as particles, that is, as objects, and then as unseen waves of energy. Whether electrons are seen or unseen depends upon the design of the experiment. If the experiment was designed to prove that atoms are physical, then that was the result the researcher obtained. If, on the other hand, one wanted to prove that particles are invisible and can be seen only by the pattern of energy they produce, one obtained that result. Electrons become like the wind, unseen, but their effect can be seen, felt, and measured. With this breakthrough, the dividing line in nature between the seen and the unseen becomes almost impossible to define.

Quantum physics acknowledges the interplay of numerous energetic forces that combine to form a whole. In this light the human being is basically a dynamic process, and health is harmony of this movement, a movement of all the dynamic processes going on in the body at any one time in response to its internal and external environments. It has been proven that 98% of 120^{28} of the atoms that are found in the body are replaced annually. It is staggering that we have all that going on in us, yet physically and mentally we appear to be solid, constant, and unchanged for extended periods of time.

Quantum physics states that every atom is more than 99% empty space and that sub-atomic particles moving at lightning speed are really just bundles of vibrating energy—or patterns of activity—which are interconnected but are never seen; however, the effect of the dynamic patterns of energy can be measured. This concept can be related to a magnet. The energy field around a magnet cannot be seen. It can be felt, however, when another magnet is near; it either attracts or repels the second magnet. So we can see the result of the dynamic energy as opposed to the dynamics of the energy itself. The arrangement of iron filings can be seen, but not the force that produces the arrangement. The same is true of the wind and other natural phenomena.

The Tiller-Einstein model attempts to mathematically describe the behavior of energy/matter at velocities beyond the speed of light in order to establish a reality base for subtle energies and subtle bodies that are beyond ordinary human perception. According to the Tiller-Einstein model the first level of energies moving faster than light velocity are the etheric frequencies of matter and energy. Matter and energy are primarily electrical in nature. Matter is composed of particles such as the electron and proton, which are electrically charged, whereas the energy/matter beyond the speed of light is electro*magnetic* in nature.

Electromagnetic Current

As strange as life energy may sound, a new medical science of energy medicine is now emerging in Western culture thanks to the research of Dr. Robert Becker, a respected orthopedic surgeon and author of *The Body Electric* and *Cross Currents* (1985). His experiments prove that the body is more than a chemical and mechanical machine, that it is also an electrical unit. Research is showing that electromagnetic energy flows along pathways bearing some resemblance to meridians. Dr. Becker has documented the existence of an underlying electromagnetic life force within the body that stimulates it to grow and heal. Becker has also found that the points along the acupuncture meridians enhance the electromagnetic current flowing in the body. It was detected that the meridians had the electrical characteristics of transmission lines, while skin not associated with meridians did not. Electromagnetic medicine may be the science that unites both Eastern and Western philosophies.

Energy

The organs of our body are made of tissues, which are made of cells, molecules, and atoms, which are all whirling, pulsating, vibrating fields of energy. Energy not only surrounds us, but also it interpenetrates the cells of our body. All matter has vibration that, in turn, has a frequency. Within the body are different energy systems. On the gross or physical level [i.e., the physical level comprising the most dense level of energy] there are the biochemical and bio-electrical networks of the body. Then there are higher energies or a life force responsible for life and creative expression. This network involves the work of the finer subtle energy systems of acupuncture meridians.

Gross energy levels are currently those that can be weighed, seen, and measured. While subtle energy levels are known to exist, the scientific technology to measure them is often lacking. Science has many times proven that subtle energies such as ultrasonics and microwaves can cause sickness; why cannot other subtle energies produce health? Why is it that many people only believe what can be seen, weighed, or measured, when even science isn't that restrictive? Science admits there is a range of sound not heard by humans and knows of a range of colors not perceived by sight. In so admitting, science moves into a broader perspective of matter as energy.

In reality the building blocks of all life are particles of energy joining together to form physical matter. We are all the same energy, coalesced in different ways to create different forms and different matter. It is simply the same energy behaving differently. In one sense we do not just take in energy; we are energy.

Energy Medicine

Acupuncture has grown in acceptance among the scientific community as a direct result of research linking acupuncture analgesia with the release of endorphins within the central nervous system. The endorphin model gave scientific theorists the first conclusive experimental evidence for acupuncture's link with known pain pathways in the brain and spinal cord.

Dr. Richard Gerber, in his book *Vibrational Medicine* (1988), cites the work of a team of Korean researchers in the 1960s headed by Professor Kim Bong Han who focused their experimental work on the acupuncture meridians of animals. "Based on many experiments, Kim concluded that the meridian system not only inter-linked within itself but appeared to interconnect with all cell nuclei of the tissues." Kim confirmed the importance of continuous meridian flow to particular organs via the deep meridian systems. Reports Gerber, "He [Kim] severed the meridian going to the liver in a frog and studied subsequent microscopic changes in the liver tissue. Shortly after severing the liver meridian, the hepatocytes enlarged and their cytoplasm became very turbid. Within three days, serious vascular degeneration took place throughout the whole liver." In addition, "Kim discovered that the formation of the acupuncture meridian system preceded the development and placement of rudimentary organs in the embryo. His work suggests that some type of information flows through the meridians to the DNA control centers of the cells, providing additional modulation to the embryologic developmental process."

In a different study with human subjects, using fMRI image equipment, Korean physicist Zang-Hee Cho, a non-believer in acupuncture, at the University of California, Irvine, conducted an experiment contrasting response by the brain to stimulation of the eye by a light flashed in front of the subject versus manipulation of acupoints on the lateral side of the foot. The points stimulated run from the small toe to the ankle [BL67, BL66, BL65, and BL60] on the bladder meridian. These points are traditionally used to treat vision problems. Much to Cho's surprise, as reported in *Discover* magazine, "he found sticking a needle into someone's foot had the very same effect as shining a light in someone's eyes. And this was not the generalized analgesic effect, produced by the primitive limbic system, that was seen in the pain studies; this was a function-specific response occurring in the brain's cortex." Up until this time it was thought by acupuncture proponents that there was little connection between the brain and various organs and that stimulating an acupoint sent a message to the targeted organ directly and did not go through the brain. "Moreover," the article continues, "the magnitude of brain activity seen on acupuncture stimulation was nearly as strong as that elicited by the flash of light."

"To eliminate the possibility of a placebo effect, Cho also stimulated a non-acupoint in the big toe. There was no response in the visual cortex." Cho noticed something else of interest. "When the activation data were graphed to show the intensity of the response over time, he saw that there were two distinct reactions among the dozen volunteers. During the acupuncture phase, some showed an increase in activity, while others showed a decrease. In other words, in some people, oxygen consumption in the brain region increased, while in others it decreased." This was attributed, by an acupuncturist, to the balancing of yin and yang.

Dr. Richard Gerber explains conventional medicine's use of energy today when he writes, "Orthodox medicine has begun to gradually explore the uses of energy for treating illness: radiation to treat cancer, or electricity to alleviate pain and shrink tumors, electromagnetic fields to stimulate fracture healing, and magnetic fields to alleviate the pain and inflammation of arthritis."

Traditional Chinese Medicine

In Traditional Chinese Medicine (TCM), which is the most widely used healing system in the world, the body is viewed from a different perspective than in conventional Western medicine. This has resulted in different thoughts and beliefs. Chinese medicine operates very much at an energy level with Chi, Blood, *Jing* (Soma/Essence), and *Shen* (Psyche/Consciousness).

Its idea of striving for the balance of energy (Chi) uses a different vocabulary to describe what is considered the dynamic energy of the body. Because of cultural restraints rather than the development and use of the vocabulary of Western science, Chinese medicine has used the vocabulary of the poet. Traditional Chinese Medicine strives to balance Chi by using a variety of techniques. Chinese medicine includes acupuncture, herbal medicine, diet, meditation, physiotherapy (*Tui Na*), exercise (*Dao In, Tai Ji Chuan*, and Eight Treasurers), the energy movement therapy of Chi *Gong*, and shamanic psychotherapy. Acupuncture is developed on the Taoist model of Chi, or energy, and its state of movement within the channels or meridians of the body. It is applied when the Chi is impeded in its proper flow—the cause of illness—in order to restore flow and health.

It is important to remember that Chinese medicine theory does not move in a linear way from proposition to proposition. Instead, the whole is always present; the Yin and Yang can only be refined, never abandoned. Traditional Chinese Medicine proceeds from the assumption that each person is a universe in miniature—the same forces that shape the macrocosm are within each of us. Chinese thinking is holographic: by observing the world we gain knowledge of a single being; each aspect of the body is reflective of the whole of which it is a part; and all the parts are connected and in constant interaction with one another. The human being is formed by the intermingling of psyche and soma, known as *Shen* and Essence.

To understand TCM requires expanding your current Western thought process to include broader concepts and other ways of thinking about the mind and body, health, and illness. The easiest way to illustrate this is to make a comparison of concepts. For instance:

Western Tradition	Eastern Tradition
The emergence of the world: Big Bang theory	Taoism begins at the same point (something arising out of nothing)—the emergence of *Wu Chi* (limitless/void/nothingness represented by an empty circle).
Medicine based on Newtonian theory of everything made up of parts (atoms)	Taoism belief is holistic; everything is one.

Newtonian model	TCM model
-Where something is located (if known) and the direction of the operating force is known. The result can be known and controlled.	-Encompasses 5 Elements, Yin/Yang, Vital Substances. -The impact of the unseen upon the visible is recognized.

Western Tradition	Eastern Tradition
Health is considered to be the absence of disease.	Health sought through the merging of the body-mind with the Tao
Disease is a condition of a particular part of the body.	Illness is a condition of the sum total of the human being.
Disease caused by bacteria; little consideration given to intangibles like joy or hope	Illness is understood as a consequence of either insufficient or obstructed Chi, Moisture, or Blood, and disturbances within or between the Organ Networks.
Treats pathology, diseases, and different parts of the body in isolation, with the intent to "cure" and/or "heal"	Study of health and life, seeks to reestablish harmonious relationships among all body functions, assists in healing but acknowledging only nature can heal and the body has the ability to heal itself
Belief in only what can be seen, weighed, and measured	Belief in unseen forces and subtle energy of Chi
Works with anatomy & physiology, chemistry, biochemistry, nerves, nerve charts, and arteries	No correspondence to anatomical maps, uses meridians and acupuncture points
Concerned with diagnosis as a means to control body function	Concerned with diagnosis as the organizing of signs and symptoms to arrive at an accurate perception of what is going on within the body
Views the body as a machine: -Brain as a computer -The heart as a pump -Organs & glands are replaceable parts -Joints as gears and levers -Stomach as a chemical beaker	Views the body as composed of Five Elements: -Fire/air (mind/thoughts/emotions) -Water/rivers (circulation/lymph) -Earth/mountain (tissue/organs/glands) -Wood/trees (spine/bones) -Metal (chemical processes of the body/ nutrition/digestion)

An expansion in one's viewpoint of life and the way of looking at the world is first necessary to understand Traditional Chinese Medicine. The second step in understanding is learning about the philosophy of Tao, which underlines TCM, to which we will now turn.

Fig. 1

DIAGRAM OF THE BASIC PREMISE
OF CREATION*

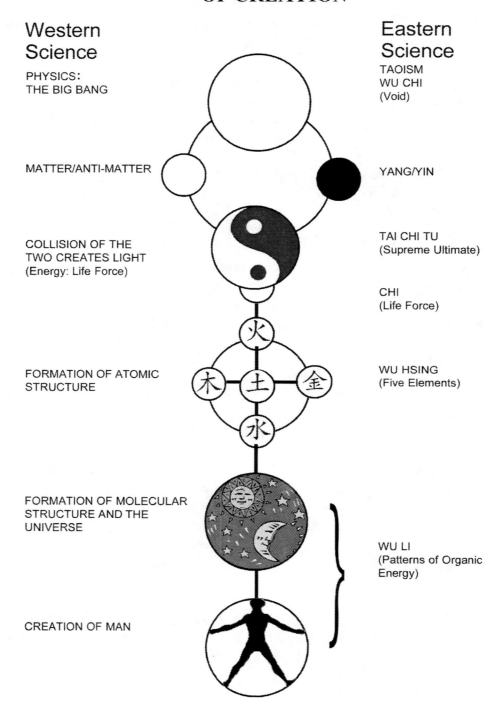

Western
Science

PHYSICS:
THE BIG BANG

MATTER/ANTI-MATTER

COLLISION OF THE
TWO CREATES LIGHT
(Energy: Life Force)

FORMATION OF ATOMIC
STRUCTURE

FORMATION OF MOLECULAR
STRUCTURE AND THE
UNIVERSE

CREATION OF MAN

Eastern
Science

TAOISM
WU CHI
(Void)

YANG/YIN

TAI CHI TU
(Supreme Ultimate)

CHI
(Life Force)

WU HSING
(Five Elements)

WU LI
(Patterns of Organic
Energy)

* Diagram adapted from work of Dr. S.C. Valentine-Marshall.

~ Chapter 2 ~

Taoist Cosmology and the History of TCM

The philosophy of the East can take a lifetime of meditation, experience, and contemplation to assimilate. However, in order to understand Chinese medicine, it is essential first to understand the basic oriental philosophy, or the Way of the Tao: the principles of life from which Traditional Chinese Medicine is derived. Briefly, Taoism describes creation based on the qualities of balance, harmony, and order among various opposing, but complementary, natural forces or energies in the macrocosm of the universe, as well as those which are reflected within the microcosm of the human being.

The Great Tao

There are two major meanings in the Chinese word *Tao*. First, Tao refers to "the Absolute-Eternal nature of all being and non-being." Second, Tao means "the Path," "the Way," or "the Road." Lao Tzu, one of the most profound Tao masters and the presumed author of the Taoist classic *Tao Te Jing,* dating back to 700 B.C.E., began with this statement: "The Tao that can be expressed in words is not the Great Tao."

While the exact meaning of the Tao cannot be explained simply by words, words can however provide us with clues that can lead us to true knowledge. Lao Tzu explains:

"Before Heaven and Earth were born,
There was something formless yet complete.
Silent! Empty!
Changeless! Hanging on nothingness!
Pervading all things! Unending!
We say it is the mother of all things under heaven,
But we do not know its real name.
We call it the Way (Tao).
We say it is Great (The Great Tao).
To be Great is to go forward,
To go forward is to travel far,
To travel far is to return,
Great is the Way,

Great are Heaven and Earth,
Great is Man.
Among the four great things,
Man follows Earth,
Earth follows Heaven,
Heaven follows the Way
The Way follows itself."

And again:

"The Great Tao is unanchored-it goes left and right.
The ten thousand creatures are nourished by it and never denied,
It creates them, and makes no demand on them.
It clothes them, but has no mastery.
So it is called humble.
So it is called great.
The Tao is hidden and nameless.
Only the Tao upholds all things
And brings them to fulfillment."

The words above have much to offer in terms of knowing oneself internally. The following phrases provide insights to understanding ourselves:

"To know people is to be wise,
To know oneself is to be illuminated.
To conquer others is to have strength
To conquer oneself is to have true power.
To be content is to have great wealth,
To follow the Way devotedly is to fulfill all aims.
Then to die and not be lost is called "long life.""

Then the question arises: where do we look in order to find the Tao?

"Many words cannot fathom it
But look, it is in your heart!"

The Tao Concepts of Change, Cycles, Oneness, Balance, and Adaptability

The Concept of Change

Tao is always manifested in Nature, and Nature itself reflects in Tao. Nothing in this world or universe is constant as Nature is in a constant state of flux. Even though sometimes some things seem to last forever, change takes place nevertheless. Eventually, everything changes, and as parameters change, "constants" must adapt. For instance, the earth, sun, and moon were born in the far distant past, exist now, and will burn out or die sometime in the future even though this cycle may take millions of years. Our life follows a similar cycle of birth to death.

According to the Tao's teaching, therefore, to hold fast to something that itself must eventually change is foolishness. Lao Tzu and the great teachers of the Tao always caution to avoid extreme attachment because attachment gives rise to rigidity. Rigidity in all things results in death while flexibility results in renewal. In the *Tao Te Jing*, Lao Tzu said, "The ancient saying 'to bend is to maintain integrity' is the word of truth."

The Concept of Cyclic Patterns

Any kind of change in nature has a process or pattern manifested as a rhythm or pulse. This cycle can be witnessed by the change in the seasons, the time, the day, and even life itself. The Chinese people took note of the cycles in the environment surrounding them. In the Chinese classic *I Ching*, or *The Book of Change,* nature's cyclical processes are recounted. The analysis in this book goes from a single cycle of change down to its sixty-four primary divisions.

As science advances, the recognition of cyclicity of all things is more pronounced. In the field of medicine, for example, the heart beats in a certain rhythm; the brain waves pulsate; and the hormones are secreted cyclically. So it is evident that every function in the body has some kind of biological rhythm or some cyclical pattern.

What does that mean to us as human beings? The Tao teaches that if we can harmonize the cycles within us with the cycles surrounding us, our life will flourish and we will be healthy both mentally and physically. The ups and downs in life, be they good or bad, will be a source of growth. Lao Tsu made the point:

"For all creatures there is a time of advancing, a time for withdrawal,
A time for inhaling, a time for exhaling,
A time for growing strong, a time for decay,
A time for creation, a time for destruction.
Therefore the wise avoid extremes and will not be lost,
Those who follow Tao avoid extremes,
Because they avoid extremes they do not expire.
They are like seeds and are constantly renewed."

The Concept of Oneness: Environment and Man are One

All things in the universe are subject to the Law of the Tao. Therefore, the Law of Nature will influence human beings. Human beings can sometimes manipulate the environment, but it is a mistake to think that we are not part of Nature or that we are superior to Nature. If we destroy the environment, eventually in return we will be destroyed. When we recognize, understand, and abide by this Law of Nature, we will treat every element of the environment with respect, as everything is one and sacred.

It is important to think of all the interrelationships of all things in the universe. Tao teaches that nothing is totally separated from everything else. Any action in anything will cause a reaction either big or small in all things. Therefore, one thing leads to another. For instance, by polluting the air we pay the consequence of breathing in unhealthy air, which ultimately can affect our health. In turn, within the body all organs and tissues play a vital part in a healthy and balanced functioning of the human body. Any disfunctioning of any cell will eventually affect the body as a whole. Chuang Tsu, another great Taoist philosopher of ancient times asks:

"In considering the human body, is it not true that its hundred bones, nine external cavities and six master organs all exist by virtue of their complete integration? May I ask which of them I shall favor the most? Should I not favor one in particular? Or is it not true that by their integration something real exists?"

The Concept of Balance

Balance is the great secret of the Tao. As long as we try to maintain balance through the ups and downs of life we will find the Tao. Conversely, having a balanced attitude and a balanced way of life smooths out the rough road of life. Bagwan Shree Rajneesh, a spiritual master, responding to the question "How can we maintain a peaceful mind in a world so tumultuous?" says:

"Who can maintain this calm for long?
Calmness comes, silence comes,
But who can maintain it for long?
By activity it comes back to life.
By activity you can maintain it.
If you try to maintain it by inactivity continuously, it will be impossible.
One has to move into opposites to remain always transcendental.
In the day you work.
In the night you sleep.
If you work continuously 24 hours, that will be death.
If you sleep 24 hours, that will be death also.
In the day work hard, and in working hard you are gaining the capacity to sleep.
In the night sleep completely, and in sleeping completely you are rejuvenating and
    refreshing your energies to work hard.
Move into a rhythm.
Lean to the right, lean to the left,
But always keep the balance...
A deep harmony.
He who embraces this Tao guards against being overful...
Then don't move too much to one side,
For the balance will be lost.
An imbalance is the only sin for Lao Tsu.
To be balanced is to be virtuous,
To be imbalanced is to be in sin.
Because he guards against being overful,
He is always fresh and young, he's never weary, he's never tired.
Balance is vitality.
Balance is Life.
Balance gives him eternal life."

The Concept of Adaptability

With all the changes, the cycles, and the Taoist way of balance in life, we must harmonize with our environment. To do so is to have the ability to adapt to any situation. According to theTao a healthy person adapts where a less adaptive person will fall and perish. The ancient Chinese recognized that the ability to adapt had to be cultivated and required the wisdom of balance. Ch'I Po, the mythical sage of *Nei Jing*, China's earliest medical text, illuminated us with three lifestyles by which ancient wise men achieved their enlightenment and immortality.

> "The ancient *Holymen* maintained their virtue and followed the Path (Tao). They lived in accord with Yin and Yang, and hence in harmony with the four seasons. They departed from the busy mundane world. They roamed the entire universe, conserving and preserving their energy with infinite freedom. In this way they strengthened and increased their life, eventually achieving immortality."

> "The ancient *Sages* attained harmony with Heaven and Earth and followed closely the Laws of Nature. They learned the art of adaptability, and thus were able to adjust their desires in order to live in harmony with all men. Without hatred or anger in their hearts, they were able to remain in the busy world. Yet they remained indifferent to the customs. They were not concerned excessively about anything. They regarded inner peace and happiness as primary, and recognized containment as the supreme achievement. They worked with their physical bodies, but avoided over-taxing themselves. They used their minds in meditation and thought, but avoided excess here as well. By following this path, they could never be harmed or depleted physically and mentally. Thus they could reach the age of one hundred years or more."

> "Then there were the men of *Supreme Virtue*. They followed Tao, obeying the laws of the universe, emulating the sun and the moon, and living by the stars. They had foresight through their observations of Yin and Yang and were thus able to move in harmony with all changes. They knew the art of harmony and lived as one within the four seasons and with all of Nature. In this way they achieved immortality."

With the understanding of the Law of the Tao, we can enhance our adaptive capacity and experience a freedom of life that can only be limited by our own weakness of will and narrowness of mind.

Historical Development of Traditional Chinese Medicine

Opposing energies were originally conceived by the emperor Fu Xi (approximately 6,000 B.C.E.) as broken and solid lines in mathematical symbolism, or as Yin and Yang. The patterns of change and transformation of various forces in Nature and in human life can be discovered through the study of the *I Ching*, or the Book of Changes, attributed to emperor Shen Nong (approximately 4,000 B.C.E.). Nong also recorded 365 plant varieties and their uses. *Shen Nong Ben Cao* is the world's oldest cohesive system of botanical knowledge. *Nei Jing* emphasizes preventive medicine through diet and influenced the development of Chinese medicine. Lao Tzu and Chuang Tzu (about 2,500 years ago) are responsible for the work, *Tao Te Jing*. This book is a reminder of a higher reality within each of us. It gives guidance for meditation and the martial arts, inspiration for healing, as well as practical wisdom for daily living, all of which are just now becoming accepted concepts within Western thought for spiritual development.

Ge Hong (283 A.D.) was a Taoist physician and alchemist whose books, *Bao Pu Zin* (on alchemy) and *Zou Hou Bei Ji Fang* (a handbook on emergency medicine), further developed the field of Chinese medicine and provided treatment for such diseases as tuberculosis, chicken pox, rabies, scrofula, and dermatological lesions. They also devised dietetic therapies for vitamin/mineral deficiency conditions such as beriberi and goiter. Taoist alchemical science was influential in the subsequent development of modern chemistry. Sun Si Miao (541 A.D.) contributed the knowledge of environmental and emotional components in the cause and treatment of disease. In his work, *Qian Jin Yo Fang*, the fields of gynecology, obstetrics, and pediatrics receive special attention. Dietetics, based on the Yin/Yang of each food was also used as the primary approach to the treatment of illness. Sun Si Miao advocated preservation of health and the uplifting of the human spirit by the return to the Tao, the harmonious, healthy way of life.

In summary it can be said that the Tao is the source of all things. It exists even before there was one. Then one begot two, representing the Polarity, Yin and Yang. Then two begot three, representing Trinity, father, mother, and son. Then three begot everything else, representing the Triad of Creation, Heaven – Life – Earth. These three are also called the Three Powers. From these three powers everything else is created. The three powers can also be the Heaven Chi, Human Chi, and Earth Chi. All lives are supported by the Heaven Chi, and without Earth Chi we cannot have life as we know it.

Whether in medicine or other Chinese arts and sciences, Taoist philosophy has been fundamental. The roots of Chinese medicine are exactly the same as those of spiritual development. By applying and sharing the simple but profound wisdom of the Tao in one's life, and through integration of Chinese medicine into complementary health care, the health of an individual and society can be improved.

In the next chapters we shall begin to delve into the various elements that make up Traditional Chinese Medicine in more detail.

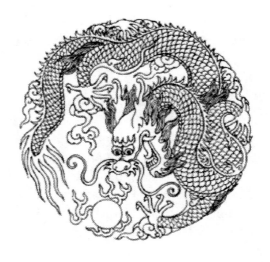

History Of Chinese Medicine

(Legendary)

1. 21st Century B.C.E.
   3494 B.C.E.   Shen-Nung - King of Farming or God of Husbandry
                                  -First pharmacologist in the world
                                  -Tasting of 100 grasses

   2674 B.C.E.   Huang Di - Yellow Emperor
                                  -*Nei Jing* (The Book of Interior)

2. 16th –11th Century B.C.E.   Used herb coating to treat diseases

3. 11th Century B.C.E.   -*Si-Jing* (book on herbs)
                                  -*San Hai Jing* (many kinds of herbs listed)
                                  -4 medical systems developed (Nutrition, Infection, Injuries,
                                   & Animal)

(Recorded History)

I   Chou

1. 541 B.C.E.   "Six Etiologies" to explain the causes of diseases

2. 407-310 B.C.E.   Pien Chueh - the first acupuncturist
                                  -*Huang Di eighty-one Nan Jing* (The Book of Medical Perplexities)

II   Ch'in

216-150 B.C.E.   Chun Yu Yi
                                  -medical case records

III   Han

1. 5 A.D.   *Shen-nong Ban Chao Jing* (Book of Herbs)

2. 112-207 A.D.   Hua Tou - first surgeon
                                  -Invented anesthesia and developed Chinese Medicine anatomy
                                  -*Five styles of boxing* (Tiger, Deer, Bear, Monkey, & Bird)

3. 196-204 A.D.   Chang Chung Ching - first medical specialist
                                  -Identification and Discussion
                                  -*Shang Han Lun* (Classic of Cold Diseases)
                                  -*Jin Kui Yao Lueh* (Golden Chest of Therapeutic Principles)

IV	Tsin	
1.	3rd Century	Wang Su Ho - pulse expert -*Mai Jing* (The Book of Pulse)

IV   **Tsin**

1. 3rd Century   Wang Su Ho - pulse expert
-*Mai Jing* (The Book of Pulse)

2. 256-282 A.D.   Huang Pu Ni - acupuncturist
-*Chia I Jing* (the earliest acupuncture book)

3. 281-341 A.D.   Ge Hong – first pharmacist
-*Zou Hou Bei Ji Fang* (handbook of emergency medicine)

4. 541 A.D.   Doctors sent to Korea by the government

5. 562 A.D.   Medical books exported to Japan

V   **Sui**

1. 608 A.D.   Doctors sent by Japan to learn Chinese medicine

2. 610 A.D.   Chao Yuan Fang – the first diagnostician of the 7th Century
Chu Ping Yuan How Lun (Cause and Symptoms of Diseases)

3. 624 A.D.   Educational department was established to teach Chinese medicine

VI   **T'ang**

1. 590-682 A.D.   Sun Szu Mo – the first formularist
Chien Chin Yao Fang (Precious Prescriptions)

2. 621-714 A.D.   Mang Sien
Shi-Liao Ban Chao (herbs used as supplements to diet)

3. 841-846 A.D.   Roung Tao Ren
-Secret method for bone realignment

4. 847-859 A.D.   Kan Yin
-*Jing Shao Chan Bo* (book on childbirth)

VII   **Sung**

1. 1026 A.D.   Wang Wei I
-The Bronze Man Acupuncture Thermocautery Drawing Book

2. 1035-1117 A.D.   Chien I - first pediatrician
-Key to Pediatric Prescriptions

3. 1102-1106 A.D.

Yang Chich Tong
-*Ts'un Chen Tu* (Anatomy Drawing Book)

4. 1103 A.D.

Central Government Pharmacy formed

5. 1107 A.D.

Chen Si Men
-Formula of Central Pharmacy

6. 1120-1200 A.D.

Liu Wan Su
-The heat origin of diseases
-Characteristics of general diseases

7. 1151-1234 A.D.

Chang Yao Shu
-Organic differential

8. 1156-1228 A.D.

Chung Tzu Ho
-Attacking therapeutic methods
-How to minister to the family

9. 1174 A.D.

Chen Yen
-Three Causes of Disease

10. 1180-1251 A.D.

Li Tung Yuan
-*Ko Chih Yu Lun* (On the Viscera)
-Identifications of internal and external diseases

11. 1186-1249 A.D.

Sung Tzu
-Forensic medicine
Si Yuam Lu
-Handling of grievance cases

12. 1281-1358 A.D.

Chu Tan Chi
-Mental diagnosis

VIII   Ming

1. 1518-1593 A.D.

Li Shih Chen - great naturalist
-*Ben Chao Kang Mu* (general catalog of herbs)

2. 1549-1613 A.D.

Wang Ken Tang
-*Liu Ko Chan Shy* (therapeutical principles of 6 departments of
general medicine, formulas, internal medicine, pediatrics,
gynecology, & injuries)

3. 1575 A.D.   Chuang Chen Pin
                                 -Ten-Question Song

4. 1592-1672 A.D.   Wu Yu Ko
                                 -Warm Diseases
                                 -The Theory of Plague

5. 1601 A.D.   Yang Chi Zhow
                                 -Great Book of Acupuncture

6. 1607-1684 A.D.   Fu Ching Chu - gynecologist
                                 -*Fu Ching Chu Nu Ca* (on gynecology and childbirth)

7. 1727 A.D.   Smallpox vaccination research, brought to England in 18th century

IX   Ch'ing

1. 1667-1746 A.D.   Yeh Tien Shih
                                 -Warm Theory
                                 -Clinical Guidance

2. 1694 A.D.   Wang Ang
                                 -Formula Song

3. 1758-1836 A.D.   Wu Ton
                                 -Differential Diagnosis of Warm Diseases

X.

18th to 19th Century   Spreading of Traditional Chinese Medicine to England, France,
                                 U.S.A., & Germany

精 氣 神 血 津 液

~ Chapter 3 ~

The Vocabulary of TCM

Every system of medicine has a language, a vocabulary of concepts, and a philosophy that establishes the criteria by which it explains itself and how it functions. Some of the most common vocabulary of TCM is defined below.

Chi / Qi	The dynamic force responsible for the activity of life, initiating movement, and the feeling of movement itself.
Congestion	Results in aches, tension, tenderness, pain, distension, irritability, and swelling.
Depletion	Leads to weakness, lethargy, frequent illness, poor digestion, and inadequate blood flow.
Disease	A disorder of relationships, not as a singular, unvarying entity.
5 Elements	Phases of being through which things tend to move. The elements themselves are Water, Wood, Fire, Earth, and Metal.
Jing / Essence	Source of life.
Meridians	Channels or pathways through which Chi moves.
Organs	The body's five main organs are the heart, lungs, kidneys, liver, and spleen. These five main organs regulate and control the body's major functions and its general health. These organs are given a great deal more power and responsibility than Western science assigns to them.
Pathology	A complex of disruptive influences upon the quantity and movement of Chi, Moisture, or Blood, all of which can become either depleted or congested.

Shen (Mind or Spirit) The vitality behind *Jing* and *Chi.*

Yin/Yang   The two basic and opposite, yet complementary, elements that make up
                     everything in the universe.

Vital (Fundamental) Substances of TCM

In TCM the body has five functional systems that govern the quantity, quality, and distribution of *Chi, Moisture, Blood,* the storage of *Essence,* and the dissemination of *Shen.* Each system refers to a complete set of functions rather than a specific physical structure fixed in an anatomical location. Because of their interconnections and interdependence, imbalance will result in the depressed function of some and hyperactivity of others. This is also stated as an excess or deficiency that in time will deteriorate into complex patterns of disharmony and disease.

Functional Systems

Essence   Represents the body's material source. The fundamental source of
(*Jing*)   regeneration and reproduction; denser energy than Blood from
                 which Blood itself is formed. We are endowed at birth with Essence,
                 part of which is replenished on a daily basis by food and air. Longevity
                 is dictated by the quality and amount of Essence.

Blood   The material foundation out of which bones, nerves, skin, muscles, and
(*Xue*)   organs are created. This energy is denser than Moisture and Chi. Blood gives
                 solidity to the shape that Chi creates. Blood is passive and tends to stagnate;
                 Chi is active and warm, which moves the Blood. Blood is the material basis
                 of Chi, linking it with physical form. They are mutually dependent upon each
                 other: where Chi goes, Blood flows, and Blood is the mother of Chi. Relative
                 to each other, Chi is more dynamic while Blood is more stable.

Moisture   The liquid medium that protects, nurtures, and lubricates tissue.
(*Jin-Ye*)   Moisture creates a buffer between tissue. This energy is denser than
                 Chi, but less so than Blood. Moisture represents a transition stage
                 between Chi and Blood.

Chi / Qi   The dynamic force responsible for the activity of life, initiating movement
                 and the feeling of movement itself. It is the animating force that provides
                 the capacity to move, think, feel, and work. This energy is less refined,
                 subtle, and intangible than *Shen.* It defines or gives things their shape. It refers
                 to the warmth and pulsatory rhythms that separate life from death.

Shen   Is associated with the immaterial expression of the individual (soul, spirit).
(Spirit)   The integrative, expressive, and self-aware aspect of mind. The least
                 tangible aspect and arises when Chi becomes self-aware. To comfort the *Shen*
                 is to soothe the spirit and relax the mind. *Shen* is responsible for this
                 integrative function and is undermined by anxiety and stress.

Shen-Jing   Refers to the totality of an individual, encompassing both the tangible and intangible realms of personal experience.

Chi, Moisture, Blood, Essence, and *Shen* are interdependent, co-generating, and mutually regulating constituents and processes. Without proper Moisture, Chi becomes hot and agitated and Blood dries up and congeals. Without Blood, Moisture is dispersed and Chi is scattered. Without Chi, both Moisture and Blood stagnate, coagulate, and stop circulating. Without Essence, the body has no material source; without *Shen,* the body lacks presence, having neither spirit nor mind.

A Closer Look at the Vital Substances

The Concept of Chi / Qi

According to the Chinese, there are many "types" of human Chi, ranging from tenuous and rarefied to dense and coarse. However, all the various types of Chi are ultimately *one* Chi, merely manifesting in different forms. Chi changes its form according to its *locality* and its *function* (e.g., Nourishing Chi vs. Protective Chi). Therefore, although it's the same Chi, clinically if either Chi is imbalanced, it is treated differently. Chi has two major aspects:

1. It indicates a refined essence produced by the internal organs. This refined essence takes several forms depending on location and function.

2. It indicates the functional activity of the internal organs. Here, it does not indicate any substance but simply the complex of functional activities of any organ.

Chi takes various forms in the body to fulfill a variety of functions. Chi is a Yang substance. It is said that everything in the universe, organic and inorganic, is composed of and defined by its Chi. TCM does not speculate on the nature of Chi, nor does it attempt to conceptualize it, but rather Chi is perceived functionally—*by what it does.*

Original Chi (*Yuan*)

It is the Essence in the form of Chi rather than fluid. It is the foundation of all the Yin and Yang energies of the body and relies on nourishment from the Post-Heaven Essence.

The four functions of original Chi are:

1. *Driving force* - The dynamic driving force that activates and moves the functional activity of all the organs. This force circulates all over the body and in the channels.
2. *Basis of Kidney Chi* - All of the Kidneys' functional activities are closely related to it.
3. *Facilitates the transformation of Chi* - It facilitates in the transformation of Chest Chi into True Chi.
4. *Facilitates the transformation of Blood* - It acts as an agent of change in the transformation of Food Chi (*Gu Chi*) into Blood in the heart.

Food Chi: *Gu Chi*, "Chi of Grains" or "Chi of Food"

After digestion, food is transformed into Food Chi by the spleen. At this stage of transformation, it is not yet in a useable form for the body. From the Middle Burner, Food Chi ascends to the Upper Burner and goes to the lungs where, combining with outside air, it forms Chest Chi. (Middle Burner and Upper Burner to be explained later in this chapter, page 27)

Note: Spleen Chi is always rising. So, if it flows down, the food is not transformed properly, and diarrhea will occur.

Chest Chi (*Zong Chi*)

In Chinese it is called "*Zong Chi*," or sometimes "Gathering Chi" or "Big Chi." The Chest Chi derives from the interaction of Food Chi with outside air. The Spleen sends Food Chi up to the Lungs where, combining with outside air, it is transformed into Chest Chi.

Functions: It controls the strength of voice and the speech, promotes and governs and directs the circulation of the Blood to the extremities.

True Chi (*Zhen Chi*)

This is the final stage of transformation of Chi in the body. Chest Chi is transformed into True Chi with the help of Original Chi. Like Chest Chi, True Chi also forms in the Lungs, hence the Lungs' function of controlling Chi in general.

Nourishing Chi (*Ying* or Nutritive Chi)

This Chi functions to nourish the internal organs and the entire body. It is closely associated with the Blood and flows within the blood vessels and in the meridians. This Chi is activated whenever a needle is inserted in or pressure is applied to an acupuncture point.

Protective Chi (*Wei Chi*)

In the Lungs where the True Chi is formed, the True Chi further divides into two forms of Chi: the refined part becomes Nourishing Chi and the crude part becomes Protective Chi. Nourishing Chi flows in the blood vessels and meridians. Protective Chi flows outside the meridians and circulates under the skin and in the flesh.

Function: To protect the body from attack by external pathogenic elements, such as Wind, Cold, Heat, and Damp.

The diagram on the following page shows the production of Chi in a person. Notice that Yuan Chi (Original Chi) is "added" to the production internally whereas all other Chi are produced externally directly or indirectly.

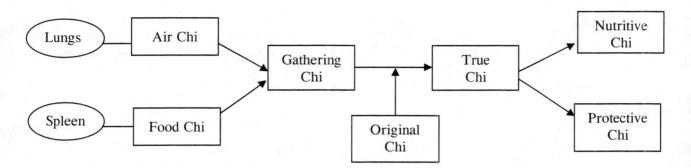

The Functions of Chi

1. Chi is the source of all movement in the body.
2. Chi protects the body.
3. Chi is the foundation of harmonious transformation in the body.
4. Chi keeps everything in.
5. Chi warms the body.

Direction of Chi Movement

Lungs: The Lungs move Chi downward.

Liver: The Liver governs the smooth flow of Chi in all directions. In particular, Liver Chi ascends.

Kidneys: The Kidneys control Water transformation, so that impure fluids descend and the clear Chi ascends. Lung Chi flows down to the Kidneys, and Kidney Chi flows up to the Lungs.

Spleen: The Spleen sends Chi upward to the Upper Burner.
Note: Upper Burner and Lower Burner to be explained later in this chapter, page 27.

Stomach: The stomach sends the impure Chi downward to the Lower Burner.

Heart-Kidneys: Heart-Fire descends to meet the water of the Kidneys, and Kidney-Water ascends to meet Heart-Fire.

Pathology of Chi

1. Chi deficient: Chi can be deficient from many factors. This is especially true for the Chi of the Spleen, Lungs, or Kidneys.

2. Chi stagnant: Chi can stagnate and be unable to move, especially Liver Chi.

3. Chi sinking: When Chi sinks, it causes prolapse of the organs. This is especially true for Spleen Chi.

4. Chi rebellious: When Chi refuses to flow in its normal direction, it is called "rebellious Chi." For example, nausea or vomiting can be the cause of Stomach Chi flowing upward instead of flowing downward.

Blood / *Xue*

Blood in TCM has a different meaning than in Western medicine. In TCM Blood is a very dense and material form of Chi, but Chi nevertheless. Moreover, Blood and Chi cannot be separated. Chi breathes life into Blood. Blood without Chi will become an inactive fluid. The main function of the Blood is to circulate continuously throughout the body, nourishing, maintaining, and moistening its different parts. Blood moves mainly through the blood vessels, but also through the Channels. Since Blood is a liquid, it is considered a Yin substance.

Source of Blood

Blood is derived from the transformation of food. The food we ingest transforms into Food Chi, which is transported up to the Lungs by Spleen Chi. When it gets to the Lungs, combining with the outside air, Blood is formed. Then the Lung Chi pushes the Blood to the Heart; then it is propelled through the body by the Heart Chi.

Fig. 3b. Production of Blood

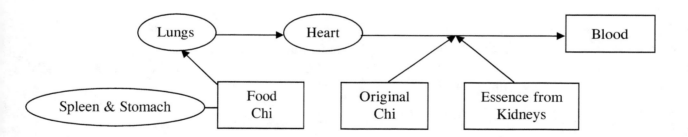

1.   The Spleen and Stomach are the main Organs that transform food to Food Chi.
2.   Lung Chi pushes Food Chi to the Heart.
3.   Blood is transformed in the Heart.

Function of Blood

1.   The main function of Blood is to nourish and moisten the body. The Blood circulates throughout the body tissues so that they do not dry out.
2.   Liver-Blood has the function of moistening the eyes, promoting good eyesight.
3.   Liver-Blood moistens tendons, promoting flexibility in joints.
4.   Liver-Blood moistens the skin as well as the hair.
5.   Heart-Blood gives the tongue its moisture.
6.   Blood houses and stabilizes the Mind (*Shen*).

Relationship with the internal organs:

Heart   *"The Heart governs the Blood."* The blood vessels are in charge of the circulation of Blood.

Spleen   Blood is originated in the Spleen as it produces Food Chi, which in term forms Blood. Spleen Chi holds Blood in the blood vessels. *"Spleen holds Blood in."*

Liver   According to TCM the Liver stores Blood. When a person is up and engaged in everyday activities, Blood flows to the muscles and tendons. When a person rests, Blood flows back to the Liver. *"The Liver stores Blood."*

Lungs   The Blood assists the Spleen in sending Food Chi to the Heart where it is transformed into Blood. Lungs control all the channels and blood vessels by infusing Chi into the blood vessels to help with the pushing action of the Heart.

Kidneys   They contribute to the production of Blood by assisting in the transformation of Food Chi into Blood, and by transforming Kidney-Essence into Blood.

Blood and Chi are mutually dependent on each other. The Chi creates and moves the Blood and also holds it in place. Blood, in turn, nourishes the organs that produce and regulate the Chi. Blood is Yin and Chi is Yang. Therefore, "Chi is the commander of the Blood and Blood is the Mother of Chi."

Pathology of Blood

1.   Blood deficiency: When Spleen Chi is weak, it causes a deficiency in the manufacturing of Blood.

2.   Blood heat: Liver-Heat can cause Blood to be hot.

3.   Blood stasis: When Blood refuses to move properly, it stagnates. This may be caused by stagnation of Liver Chi, by Heat, or by Cold.

Moisture or Body Fluids / *Jin-Ye*

Body Fluids are called *Jin-Ye* in Chinese. "*Jin*" means "moist" or "saliva," and "*Ye*" means "fluid."

"*Jin*" indicates anything that is liquid—lighter and clearer fluids—while "*Ye*" refers to fluids with a heavier and thicker nature, fluids of living organisms (that are found in plants, for instance). Thus, *Jin-Ye* is sometimes referred to as "organic fluids." In TCM, Body Fluids refer to bodily liquids other than Blood, including sweat, saliva, gastric juices, tears, and urine.

Source

Body Fluids are derived from food and drink. Spleen transforms and separates the Fluids: a "clean" part is sent from the Spleen to the Lungs, which spread a portion of it to the skin and send a portion of it down to the Kidneys. A "dirty" part is sent down to the Small Intestine where again it is divided into pure and impure portions. The "pure" portion of this second separation goes to the Bladder, and the "impure" portion descends down to the Large Intestine, where some water is re-absorbed. The Bladder further transforms and divides the fluids into a pure and impure portion. The pure portion ascends and flows to the exterior of the body where sweat is formed. The impure portion descends and is transformed into urine.

Kidney-Yang is responsible for producing the Chi that assists the Bladder in this function of transformation and separation. This function of the Bladder is called "function of Chi transformation." The Fluids depend on the Chi, and the Chi, to some extent, depends on the Fluids to moisten and nourish the Organs that regulate Chi.

Types of Body Fluids:

Fluids are *Jin*

These clear fluids are light and thin-watery and circulate with Protective Chi on the exterior (skin and muscles). They move relatively fast. They moisten and partially nourish the skin and muscle. Examples of clear fluids are sweat, tears, saliva, and mucus. The fluids also are a component of the fluid part of Blood.

Liquids are *Ye*

These fluids are cloudy, heavy, and dense. They circulate relatively slowly with Nourishing Chi in the interior. They moisten the joints, spine, brain, and bone marrow. *Ye* also lubricate the eyes, ears, nose, mouth, and other orifices of the sense organs.

Function of Fluids

The function of the Body Fluids is to moisten and partly to nourish the hair, skin, membranes, flesh, muscles, inner organs, orifices, brain, marrow, joints, and bones.

Relationship with the Internal Organs

Spleen

The Spleen governs the beginning stage of transformation and separation into a pure and impure part. It also directs the pure and impure parts upward and downward respectively at all stages of Body Fluids' production. In TCM, the Spleen is treated in any type of disorders of Body Fluids.

Lungs

The Lungs have the ability to disperse the pure portion of Body Fluids coming from the Spleen to the flesh under the skin. This is the Lung-dispersing-function aspect. The Lungs also send a portion of the fluids down to the Kidneys and Bladder. This is the Lung-descending-function aspect.

Kidneys

They transform the fluids into a "mist" form and send them back up to the Lungs to moisten the Lungs and prevent them from becoming too dry. Kidney-Yang is important in that it controls many stages of the transformation of fluids. The Kidneys:

1. Provide the heat crucial for the Spleen to transform Body Fluids.
2. Assist the Small Intestine's function to separate Body Fluids into a pure and impure part.
3. Provide Chi to the Bladder's function of Chi transformation.
4. Assist the Triple Burner (See below) in transforming and excreting Body Fluids.

Bladder

Chapter 3 of *The Foundations of Chinese Medicine* by Giovanni Maciocia says: *"The Bladder separates the fluids it receives into a pure and impure part and it excretes urine by the power of Chi transformation."*

The Triple Burner

In TCM, the Triple Burner comprises "areas" that are defined by specific energy concepts, which have no or little correspondence to actual physical organs known to Western medicine. The term Triple Burner is interchangeable with Triple Warmer and Triple Heater.

The Triple Burner consists of the Upper, Middle, and Lower Burners. They aid in the transformation, transportation, and excretion of Body Fluids at all stages. The Upper Burner, called "mist," assists the Lungs in dispersing them to the flesh under the skin. The Middle Burner, called "muddy pool," assists the Spleen's function in directing the pure fluids upwards and the Stomach's function of churning the fluids and directing the impure part downwards. The Lower Burner, known as "drainage ditch," assists the Small Intestine, Bladder, and Kidneys in their functions of transforming, separating, and excreting fluids.

Stomach

The Fluids first enter the Stomach from where they are transformed and separated with the assistance of the Spleen. The Stomach likes to be relatively moist, whereas the Spleen likes to be dry and can be damaged by too much dampness.

Pathology of Body Fluids

1. Deficiency of Body Fluids is seen in the form of dryness occurring on the lips, eyes, etc.
2. Accumulation of Body Fluids is seen in the form of edema or phlegm-fluids.

Essence / *Jing*

Essence is the substance that underlies all organic life. It is the source of organic change. It is fluid-like and is supportive and nutritive. And it is the basis of reproduction and development. It is a precious substance to be cherished and guarded within the human body. It is a denser form of Chi.

The differences between Essence and Chi:

1. Essence is primarily derived before birth from parents, and Chi is mostly formed after birth.
2. Essence is more substantial and fluid-like; Chi is non-substantial and energy-like.
3. Essence is stored mostly in Kidneys; Chi is all over.
4. Essence takes a long time and is difficult to replenish. Chi can be replenished on a daily basis.
5. Chi can move and change instantly. Essence changes gradually and slowly over long periods of time.

There are three forms of Essence:

Prenatal (Pre-Heaven) Essence

Conception is a unification of the sexual energies of a man and woman to form *Prenatal Essence* of the newly conceived human being. Essence is passed on from the parents to the embryo at time of conception. The *Prenatal Essence* along with the mother's Kidneys nourishes the embryo and fetus during pregnancy. The quality and quantity of *Prenatal Jing* are mostly fixed at birth and, together with Original Chi, determine a person's basic makeup, constitution, strength, and vitality. It's what makes each person unique. *Pre-Heaven Essence* can be depleted by the imbalance of work and rest, too much sexual activity, and bad diet. It can be positively influenced, however, through breathing exercises, e.g., *Tai Ji Chuan* or Chi *Gong*.

Postnatal (Post-Heaven) Essence

Postnatal Essence is refined and extracted from food and fluids by the Stomach and Spleen after birth. It is derived from the purified parts of ingested food and fluids. It constantly adds vitality to the *Prenatal Jing*.

Kidney-Essence

Kidney-Essence is a more specific kind of energy that is very important in the human physiology. It partakes of both *Pre-* and *Post-Heaven Essences*. It determines growth, reproduction, development, sexual maturation, conception, and pregnancy. *Kidney-Essence* is stored in the Kidneys but, having a fluid nature, it circulates all over the body.

Functions and Pathology of Essence

An individual's development is accompanied by corresponding changes in his or her *Jing*. The *Nei Jing* speaks of women's development in *seven-year* stages and of men's in *eight-year* stages.

1. Reproduction, growth, and development

Essence's function is to control the growth of bones in children, teeth, hair, normal brain development, and sexual maturation. After puberty, it governs the reproductive function and fertility. Therefore, if Essence is depleted, it will result in decline of sexual energy and fertility. Deficiency results in stunted growth in children, poor bone development, infertility, habitual miscarriage, mental retardation in children, bone deterioration in adults, loose teeth, and hair falling out or graying prematurely.

2. Essence as basis of Kidney Chi

There are four closely interacting aspects of the kidney energy:

Kidney-Essence;
Kidney-Yin;
Kidney-Yang; and
Kidney Chi.

Kidney-Essence along with the warming action of Kidney-Yang is essential in transforming Kidney-Yin into Kidney Chi. Deficiency of Essence results in poor sexual function, impotence, weakness of knees, nocturnal emissions, tinnitus, and deafness.

3. Essence produces Marrow

Different from Western medicine, it does not correspond to bone marrow. In TCM Essence produces Marrow, which in turn produces bone marrow and fills the spinal cord and the brain. Deficiency of Essence results in poor concentration, poor memory, dizziness, tinnitus, and feeling of emptiness of the head.

4. Essence as the basis of constitutional strength

Essence determines the basic constitutional strength and resistance to external pathogenic factors. A deficiency results if one is constantly prone to colds, influenza and other exterior diseases, chronic rhinitis, and hay fever.

Essence and Chi are also the material foundation of the Mind (*Shen*). In TCM the *Three Treasures* are *Essence, Chi,* and *Mind*, which represent three different states of the condensation of Chi.

Densest:	Essence (*Jing*)
Rarefied:	Chi
Subtlest and immaterial:	Mind (*Shen*)

If Essence and Chi are healthy and thriving, the Mind will be content and this will lead to a healthy and happy life. If Essence and Chi both are depleted, the Mind will suffer. The triad of Essence, Chi, and Mind is expressed in TCM as:

Mind	-	Heaven	-	Heart
Chi	-	Person	-	Stomach/Spleen
Essence	-	Earth	-	Kidneys

Imbalance of *Jing*

Jing is the source of life. Improper maturation, sexual dysfunction, inability to reproduce, and premature aging are the signs of imbalanced *Jing*. The congenital defects that are known to the West often are considered *Jing* irregularities in TCM.

Spirit / *Shen*

Shen is the vitality and consciousness behind *Jing* and Chi in the human body. *Shen* is associated with the human personality, the ability to think, discriminate, and choose appropriately, or, as is commonly said: "*Shen is the awareness that shines out of our eyes when we are truly awake.*" *Shen* does not have a material aspect, yet it is as much a part of the body as the stomach.

Origin of *Shen*

Like the origin of *Jing*, parents create their offspring's *Shen*, yet the *Shen* is also continuously and materially nourished after birth from food and drink. A healthy person's *Shen* is the capacity of the mind to form ideas and is the aspiration of the personality to live life.

Imbalance of *Shen*

A person's eyes may lack luster; he or she may not be thinking clearly, and sometimes even be mentally confused. Other signs are slow, forgetful, incoherent speech. In extreme cases the individual may be unconscious or violently angry.

Shen	-Greater Yang	*Jing*	-Greater Yin
Chi	-Lesser Yang	Blood	-Lesser Yin

Adverse Body Climates

Cold, Heat, Wind, Dampness, and Dryness

Heat	Symptoms of inflammation (internal heat)
Cold	Symptoms of shivers, regardless of external temperature (lowered metabolic activity)
Dampness	Symptoms of swelling and sense of fullness, heaviness, and lethargy (excess moisture)
Dryness	Symptoms of dehydration (lack of moisture)
Wind	Can create the pre-conditions for Dampness, Dryness, Cold, and Heat
Wind-Cold	Chills, body aches, and clear, runny secretions
Wind-Heat	Fever, thirst, stuffy nose, and yellow secretions
Wind-Damp	Can obstruct the nerves and sense organs—neurological disorders

Wind-Water   Can create swelling, such as edema on the face, cough with white and watery mucus, sweating, no thirst, floating pulse

The complementary principle can generally be used: for Cold, apply warmth; for Heat, coolness; for congested Chi, Moisture, or Blood, encourage movement; for depletion, nourish; for Internal Wind, subdue; for External Wind, relieve surface congestions; and for phlegm, dissolve.

Having defined a few of the most common words of TCM that explain its characteristic actions and the five functional systems that govern the quantity, quality, and distribution of Chi, we turn to the next task of refining other basic concepts of Yin and Yang, the Internal Organs, the Five Elements, the meridians, and the acupuncture points over the next several chapters.

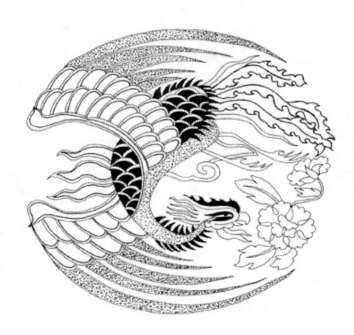

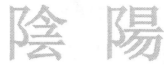

~ Chapter 4 ~

Theory of Yin and Yang

The whole of Traditional Chinese Medicine can be reduced to the basic and fundamental theory of Yin and Yang. In TCM emphasis is placed on the concept of balance and the balance between two basic and opposite, yet complementary, elements of Yin and Yang that make up everything in the universe. Yin is a negative or passive element, and Yang is a positive or active element. No judgment is attached with either element. They are dependent on each other, for there can be no night without day, no hot without cold, no joy without sorrow. Western dualism has the concept of opposites. However, the concept is different in TCM. It is about a relationship. Yin and Yang are opposites in that they depend on each other because they only exist in relationship with their opposite. Yin and Yang form a whole.

Nature of Yin and Yang Concept

The Yin-Yang symbol represents the way things change. Each part has a dot of the opposite color in its center, representing two poles that contain at their innermost core the essence of the opposite, reminding us that nothing is merely Yin or Yang. The Chinese characters for Yin and Yang are related to the dark and sunny sides of hills.

Fig. 4a.
Symbol of Tao, Representing Yin &Yang

Yin (▼)	Yang (Δ)
Shady side of the hill	Sunny side of the hill
Moon	Sun
Matter	Energy
Earth	Heaven
Night	Day
Cold	Hot
Negative	Positive
Female	Male
Contraction	Expansion

Continuation of Yin and Yang pairings:

Yin (▼)	Yang (Δ)
Inhalation	Exhalation
Autumn	Spring
Winter	Summer
Lower	Upper
Front	Back
Interior/Deep	Exterior/Surface
Water	Fire
Soft and receptive	Hard and unyielding
Quiet	Noise
Substance	Function
Dim	Bright

Cycles

Yin and Yang are the two phases of a cyclical movement, that is, one is constantly changing into the other, and vice versa.

Yin (▼)	Yang (Δ)	
Night	Day	Two stages of a cyclical
Rest	Activity	movement, one constantly
Darkness	Light	changing into the other,
Moon	Sun	and vice versa.
Shade	Brightness	
Earth	Heaven (where the sun is)	* Based on the
Space	Time	Chinese calendar,
Flat/Square	Round	Heaven is time and
West	East	Earth is space.
North	South	
Right	Left	

*Heaven is a pure, gas-like state; Earth is a dense material, a coarse and solid state.

Yin and Yang as two phases of a cyclical movement are expression of a duality in time, an alternation of two opposite stages in time. In addition, all phenomena alternate through a cycle of peaks and valleys—day changes into night, summer into winter, growth into decay, etc. The daily cycle illustrates the changes of Yin and Yang.

Fig. 4b. Symbols Representing Four Segments of a Day

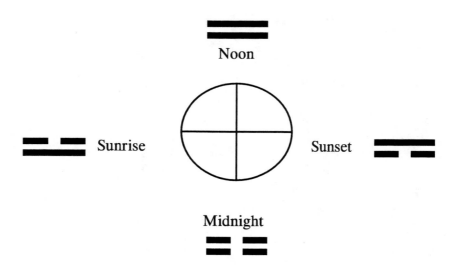

The two intermediate stages do not represent neutral stages, because they still pertain primarily to one or the other, i.e., dawn/spring is Yang; dusk/autumn is Yin. The yearly cycles of seasons—spring, summer, autumn, winter—act in the same manner.

Yin and Yang as two stages of transformation:

Yin (▼)	Yang (△)
Material	Immaterial
Cloud	Rain
Produces form	Produces energy
Substantial	Non-substantial
Matter	Energy
Contraction	Expansion
Descending	Rising
Below	Above
Water	Fire
Downward	Upward
Standstill	Moving

The Five Fundamental Principles of Yin and Yang Theory

Although they are opposite stages, Yin and Yang form a unity and are complementary to each other.

1. All Things Have Two Aspects: Yin and Yang. Nothing in the natural world escapes this opposition, yet it is relative, not absolute, as nothing is totally Yin or Yang. The two aspects are dynamic and constantly changing toward balance.

2. Each Aspect Can Be Further Subdivided Into Yin and Yang. For example, Hot is Yang relating to Cold; Boiling relating to Lukewarm; or using Western medicine, distal to proximal.

3. Yin and Yang Create Each Other, just as the chicken is Yang and the egg is Yin, but both are two aspects of the same thing.

4. Yin and Yang Mutually Define Each Other. There can be no night without day. This is not a cause-and-effect relationship. It is a circular relationship between the two.

5. At Their Extremes, Yin and Yang Transform Into Each Other, that is, when anything reaches its extreme, it becomes completely its opposite. For example, if you throw a ball upward, at some point it ceases upward movement and falls back to the ground. At a certain stage of development, all things can change from Yin to Yang, and vice versa: day into night, life into death, happiness into unhappiness, heat into cold, etc.

Application of Yin and Yang to Chinese Medicine

Health is the balance of Yin and Yang. Any illness can be explained according to the concept of the Five Elements. In TCM the Yin and Yang phases of the illness must be known before it can be treated effectively through the balancing of Yin and Yang. Ultimately, every treatment aims to:

1. Tonify Yang
2. Tonify Yin
3. Eliminate excess Yang or
4. Eliminate excess Yin

Fig. 4c. Diagrammatic representations of balance and imbalances of Yin and Yang

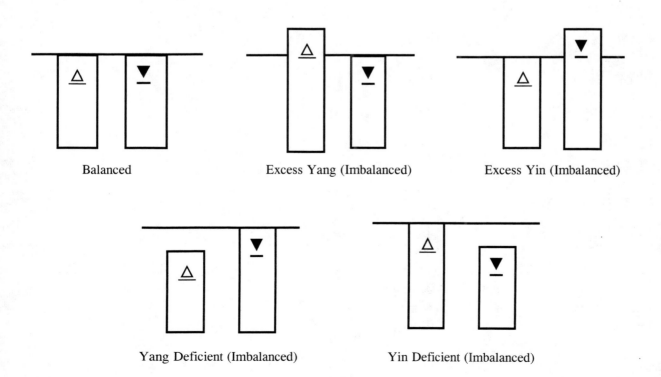

Balanced   Excess Yang (Imbalanced)   Excess Yin (Imbalanced)

Yang Deficient (Imbalanced)   Yin Deficient (Imbalanced)

Body Structure vs. Yin and Yang

Yin (▼)	Yang (Δ)
Front (Anterior)	Back (Posterior)
Body	Head
Interior (Organs)	Exterior (Skin/Muscles)
Below Waist (Inferior)	Above Waist (Superior)
Yin Organs	Yang Organs (Bowels)
Structure of Organs	Functions of Organs
Blood/Body Fluids	Chi
Nourishing Chi	Protective Chi

Yin and Yang in Anatomy and Physiology

Yin (▼)	Yang (Δ)
(Organs)	**(Organs/Bowels)**
Heart	Small Intestine
Liver	Gall Bladder
Lungs	Large Intestine
Kidneys	Bladder
Spleen	Stomach
Pericardium	Triple Burner (Triple Warmer)
(Body Parts)	
Interior	Exterior
Abdomen/Front	Spine/Back
Lower Body	Upper body
(Tissues)	
Bones	Surface Skin
Tendons	Body Hair
(Activity and Function)	
Blood and Fluids	Chi and Defense
Rest	Activity
Recovery	Metabolism
Depression	Excitation
Regression	Progression
Hypo	Hyper

Yin (▼)	Yang (Δ)

(Disease)

Yin (▼)	Yang (Δ)
Interior	Exterior
Deficiency	Excess
Cold	Heat

Yin/Yang Associations

Yin (▼)	Yang (Δ)

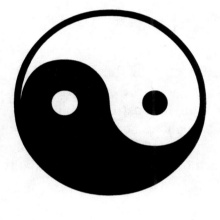

Yin	Yang
Matter	Energy
Dark	Light
Female	Male
Earth	Heaven
Hard	Soft
Lower	Higher
Inner	Outer
Consolidating	Expanding
Cold	Hot
Winter	Summer
Moon	Sun
Organs	Bowels

Taiji Tu

臟 腑

~ Chapter 5 ~

The Internal Organs of the Body

In TCM it is taught that the body's five main Internal Organs are the Heart, Lungs, Kidneys, Liver, and Spleen. These five main organs regulate and control the body's major functions and its general health. The functions of the Internal Organs are to produce, maintain, replenish, transform, and move the Vital Substances. Each of the Vital Substances is related to one or more of the organs. Therefore:

The Heart governs the Blood and stores *Shen*.
The Liver stores Blood and makes sure the Chi spreads smoothly all over the body.
The Lungs rule Chi and influence Body Fluids.
The Spleen governs the Food Chi, manages Blood, and influences Body Fluids.
The Kidneys govern Essence and influence Body Fluids.

The inner organs are interpreted more as a body-mind-spirit unit than as anatomical forms with physiological functions. Thus, each organ makes a contribution to the whole personality, and its interactions with other organs are of utmost importance to the mental and emotional levels. Organs are not looked upon from a physiological standpoint but as an expression of the five elemental forces and their constant interplay (more like our body systems rather than the individual organs for which they are named).

In Chinese the Internal Organs are called the *Zang Fu*. These organs are given a great deal more power and responsibility than Western science assigns to them. All the remaining organs are secondary to them and largely controlled by them.

Each of the Internal Organs contains an element of Yin and Yang although each contains more of one than the other. Chi, or the vital force, which is thought to be inherent in all things and among the *Zang Fu* organs, controls the balance of Yin and Yang in the body. In the healthy body, the Yin and Yang properties within are constantly fluctuating yet remain in continuous balance with each other. When Yin and Yang go out of balance, poor health generally follows.

The food eaten can disrupt the balance in the body. In TCM when the food leaves the stomach, the elements of that food are directed to certain organs based on the taste value of the particular food. Sour foods go to the liver; bitter foods go to the heart; sweet foods go to the spleen; pungent foods go to the lungs; and salty foods go to the kidneys. Through proper food selection, combining, and preparation it is possible to balance the Yin and Yang of foods.

There are two types of Internal Organs: Yin (called "*Zang*") and Yang (called "*Fu*") organs.

Zang means organ. The Chinese character of "Zang" means "flesh" that "stores."

Therefore, Yin organs are in charge of storing the Vital Substances of Chi, Blood, Essence, Body Fluids, and *Shen*. They only store pure, refined substances that are received from the Yang organs after transformation from food. These are physically the more "solid" organs.

Fu also means organ. The Chinese character of "Fu" means "flesh" that has the "seat of governing."

The Yang organs do not store but are constantly filled and emptied. The Yang organs are referred to as Yang Bowels. Anatomically these organs are "hollow." The Yang organs control the transformation of food and drink to produce Chi and Blood. They transform and refine food and drink to extract the pure essences that are then stored by the Yin organs. The functions of the Yang organs are to receive, move, transform, digest, and excrete waste products.

Yin Organs	Yang Bowels
Heart	Small Intestine
Liver	Gall Bladder
Lungs	Large Intestine
Spleen	Stomach
Kidneys	Bladder
Pericardium	Triple Burner

The Yin Organs

The Heart (*Xin*) The King Organ

In TCM it is said, *"The Heart governs the Blood and Blood Vessels."* The flow of the Blood depends on the Heart, and Blood flows smoothly when the Heart is functioning properly. If the Blood and Chi of the Heart are abundant and normal, then the pulse will be even and regular.

"The Heart houses the Shen." When there is harmony in the Heart's Blood and Chi, *Shen* is nourished and the individual can respond to the environment appropriately. When the *Shen* is not stored properly, the individual may show signs like insomnia, excessive dreaming, or forgetfulness. In the more serious disorders, symptoms like hysteria, irrational behavior, insanity, and delirium may occur.

"The Heart opens to the tongue." The Heart's Blood and Chi are closely related to the tongue, and the tongue can show any disorder of the Heart. Usually a pale tongue indicates deficient Blood in the Heart. Also, a purplish tongue shows stagnation of the Heart Blood.

"The Heart manifests in the complexion." If the Heart Blood is plentiful, one's face has a normal reddish complexion and will be moist and bright. However, if the Heart Blood is insufficient, one's face will be pale and without luster. If the Heart Blood is stagnant, one's face may be purplish. Too much redness in the complexion indicates there is too much Heart Heat. Dry skin may show that the Heart is weak. Rashes show that the Heart is trying to get rid of toxins; the Blood is toxic.

"The Heart controls sweat." Sweat as one of the Body Fluids comes from the space between skin and muscles. Since Blood and Body Fluids mutually interchange, and the Heart governs Blood, then the Heart is related to sweat. Deficiency of Heart Chi results in spontaneous sweating, and deficiency of Heart Yin can cause night sweating. Treat the former case by tonifying Heart-Yang and the latter case by tonifying Heart-Yin. "To tonify" means to activate, to increase, to add, or to boost Chi.

"Dreams are related to the heart." Since the Heart controls the *Shen* (Mind), it is directly related to sleep. If the Heart is strong, the *Shen* resides in the Heart, and one will fall asleep easily and sleep soundly. If the Heart is weak, the Mind will "float" at night, causing failure to sleep, disturbed sleep, or excessive dreaming. All dreams are related to the Heart.

The Lungs (*Fei*)

The *Nei Jing* calls the Lungs "the Lid of the Yin Organs" due to the fact that they form a cap or lid on top of all the other Organs. The Lungs are called the "tender organs" because they are the Yin organs most easily affected by external influences. The Lungs direct Chi in descending and circulating movements.

"The Lungs governs the Chi." Through respiration, the Lungs, in a sense, control the Chi of the entire body. The Lungs are where the outside Chi meets with the Chi of the body. The Lungs take in outside air/Chi by the "descending" property, thus inhalation. Exhalation takes place when the Lungs push the impure air outward. When the Lungs are healthy, air can enter and leave smoothly, and respiration will be even and regular. Imbalance of the Lungs results in symptoms like cough, asthma, and chest distention.

"The Lungs regulate water passage." The Lungs have a role in the movement and transformation of water in the body. The Lungs liquefy water vapor and move it down to the Kidneys via the descending property. The Lungs "circulate" the water vapor throughout the body, particularly through the skin and pores. The Lungs are also known as "the upper origin of water." Disharmony in the "descending" function of the Lungs results in problems of urination and edema in the upper part of the body. Disharmony in the circulating function of the Lungs results in perspiration problems.

"The Lungs govern the exterior of the body." The Lungs regulate the secretion of sweat, the moistening of the skin, and resistance to the external influences. These functions depend on the Protective (*Wei*) Chi, which in turn depends on the Lungs' circulating function. If Lung Chi is weak, there may be too much or too little sweat and the resistance of *Wei* Chi is poor.

"The Lungs' brilliance is manifested in the body hair." This means that the quality of the body hair indicates the condition of the Lung Chi.

"The Lungs opens into the nose." The nose is the opening of the Lungs, and through it respiration occurs. If Lung Chi is strong, the nose will be open, respiration will be easy, and sense of smell normal. If Lung Chi is weak, the Lungs can be attacked by the exterior pathogenic factor, the nose will be clogged up, and there may be loss of the sense of smell and sneezing. If Lungs have heat, there may be bleeding from the nose.

The Spleen (*Pi*)

The Spleen is the central organ of digestion according to the Chinese. It is called the *"Granary official from whom the five tastes are derived."*

"The Spleen governs transformation and transportation." The Spleen is responsible for the transformation of Blood and Chi from food in the process of digestion. The Spleen Chi sends the *Gu Chi*, derived from food and the "pure essences" that will become Blood, upward to the Lungs. The Spleen is also involved in the movement and transformation of Water in the body. If the Spleen Chi is sufficient and harmonious, the Chi and Blood will be abundant and the digestive powers strong. If the Spleen is in disharmony, the body may suffer from Chi or Blood deficiency. If digestion is affected, symptoms like abdominal distention or pain, diarrhea, or anorexia may appear.

"The Spleen controls the Blood." The Spleen Chi keeps the Blood flowing in its proper paths by holding the Blood in place. If the Spleen Chi is weak, the Spleen controlling function loses its harmony, and the Blood will escape its pathways and "move recklessly." The results are vomiting blood, blood in stool, blood under skin, or uterine bleeding.

"The Spleen controls the muscles and the four limbs." The Spleen transports the Chi and Blood to the muscles and skin. The movement of the muscles, skin, and the four limbs depends on the power of the Spleen.

"The Spleen opens into the mouth and manifests in the lips." The mouth and lips are strongly related to the Spleen. If the Spleen is healthy, the mouth will be able to distinguish the five tastes of bitter, sour, sweet, salty, and spicy/pungent. The lips will be red and moist. If the Spleen is not strong, the mouth will not be sensitive to taste and the lips will be pale and lifeless.

The Liver (*Gan*)

The Liver has many vital functions in the body, including storing the Blood and ensuring the smooth flow of Chi throughout the body.

"The Liver ensures the smooth flow of Chi." The Liver moves the Chi and Blood in all directions, sending them to every part of the body. The *Nei Jing* calls the Liver "the general of an army" because it makes sure that the Chi movement flows smoothly throughout the body. If the Liver is in disharmony, the Chi of the body stagnates.

"The Liver stores Blood." The Liver stores and regulates the Blood. According to the traditional thinking: when one moves, the Blood moves to the Meridians; and when one rests, the Blood returns to the Liver. When in disharmony, the Liver stores the Blood insufficiently, resulting in not enough Blood to nourish the eyes, making them rough and dry. If the Liver is not able to store the Blood, it manifests itself as an unusually heavy menstrual flow.

"The Liver rules the tendons and is manifest in the nails." When Liver Blood is plentiful, the tendons are supple and flexible and the nails appear pink and moist. When in disharmony, spasms, numbness of the limbs, and difficulty in bending or stretching may occur. Thin, brittle, and pale nails can indicate Liver disharmony.

"The Liver opens into the eyes." The *Nei Jing* says, "When the Liver is harmonized, the eyes can distinguish the five colors (of white, yellow, red, blue-green, and black)," and "When the Liver receives Blood, the eyes can see." Apart from the Liver, other Yin and Yang organs that affect the eyes are the Heart, Kidneys, Lungs, Gall Bladder, Bladder, and Small Intestine.

The Kidneys (*Shen*)

The Kidneys, the "Root of Life," or the "Root of the Pre-Heaven Chi," store the Essence that is partly from the parents and established at conception.

"The Kidneys store the Jing." The Kidneys govern birth, development, and maturation. The Essence is the source of life and affects individual development. Ultimately, the Yin and Yang, or the life activity, of each Organ depends on the Yin and Yang of the Kidneys, thus the saying of the Kidneys as the "Root of Life."

"The Kidneys govern Water." The Kidney-Yang fire transforms Water into a "mist," a necessary first step before sending the Fluids upward or in circulation. The process of Water movement will be smooth if the Kidneys are harmonious.

The Web That Has No Weaver, Chapter Three, says, "The system of Water movement may be summarized as follows. Fluids are received by the Stomach, which begins a process of separation, by which the unusable portions of food are sent to the intestines as waste and the pure Water is extracted. This process is continued by the Spleen, which then sends the pure Fluids in a vaporized state upward to the Lungs. The Lungs circulate the clear part of the Fluids throughout the body, but liquefy whatever has become impure through use and send it downward to the Kidneys. In the Kidneys, the impure part is further separated into relatively "clean" and "turbid" parts. The clear part is transformed into a mist and sent upward to the Lungs, where it rejoins the cycle. The final impure portion goes into the Bladder, where it is stored and subsequently excreted."

"The Kidneys rule the bones and produce the marrow." The marrow, which is responsible for creating and supporting bones, is produced by the Kidney *Jing*. The development and repair of bones depend on the nourishment of the Kidney *Jing*.

"The Kidneys open into the ear." The relationship between the Kidneys and the ears is very close. According to *Nei Jing*, "The Kidney Chi goes through the ear; if the Kidney is harmonized, the ears can hear the "five tones.""

"The Kidneys manifest in the head hair." The Kidney *Jing* controls the relative moistness and vitality of head hair. Loss of hair due to aging shows the weakness of Kidney *Jing*. Premature graying of the hair indicates stress in or depletion of Kidney Chi/Essence.

"The Kidneys control the reception of Chi." The Lungs and Kidneys work together for making use of the "pure Chi" of the outside air. Lungs descend the air to the Kidneys whose function is to hold the Chi down. If the Kidneys are too weak to hold the Chi, breathlessness and asthma may occur. This is usually the cause of chronic asthma.

Pericardium *(Xin-Bao)*

Many of the functions of the Pericardium are the same as the functions of the Heart. Since it forms the exterior of the Heart, it has the function of protecting the Heart from external pathogenic factors. However, in TCM the Pericardium is of secondary importance to the Heart. Many of the acupuncture points on the Pericardium Channel have influences on the mental and emotional state of the person. Moreover, the Pericardium Channel itself is very distinct from the Heart Channel and has a different sphere of action, influencing the area at the center of the thorax.

The Yang Bowels

The Stomach *(Wei)*

Of all the Yang Organs, the Stomach is the most important one. Together with the Spleen, it is called the "Root of the Post-Natal Chi" due to the fact that it is the origin of all the Chi and Blood produced after birth.

The function of the Stomach, as the origin of fluids, is to control:

the "rotting and ripening" of food;
the transportation of food essences; and
the descending of Chi.

It is called the "sea of food and fluids." Food decomposes in the Stomach. The "pure" part is transported to the Spleen. The Spleen transforms the "pure" part into the raw material for Chi and Blood. The "dirty" part is transported to the Small Intestine for more digestion. Stomach and Spleen work closely together. The Spleen Chi ascends, and the Stomach Chi descends. Disorder of the Stomach's function of descending will cause symptoms like nausea, stomachache, distention, belching, or vomiting.

The Stomach has an effect on the mental state of the person. The Stomach can easily suffer from Excess patterns (Fire). This will cause one closing off from the world, shutting oneself in the house, wanting to be alone, uncontrolled talking, laughing, or singing, violent behavior, taking off of one's clothes—manic behavior. Also Stomach-Fire can cause mental confusion, severe anxiety, hypomania, and hyperactivity.

The Small Intestine *(Xiao Chang)*

Receiving and separating food and fluids are the roles of the Small Intestine. The Small Intestine further separates the pure part from the impure part. It continues the process of separation and absorption of what comes from the Stomach. Again the pure part extracted by the Small Intestine is sent to the Spleen, and the impure part is sent downward to the Large Intestine. At this point of separation of parts, some impure fluid is also sent directly to the Kidneys and Bladder. Disorder of the Small Intestine will cause abdominal pain, intestinal rumbling, diarrhea, or constipation.

Although the Heart is the Yin Organ of the Small Intestine according to the 5-Element theory, there is not a very close relationship between the two in relation to functions. The closest tie between these two organs is found on the psychological level. The Heart houses the *Shen,* and the Small Intestine influences the mental clarity, judgment, and one's capacity to make decisions. If deficient, one cannot make a decision because one cannot see any other option and therefore cannot make the right choice.

The Large Intestine *(Da Chang)*

Receiving food and drink from the Small Intestine is the major role of the Large Intestine. Then the Large Intestine excretes the stools after re-absorbing some of the fluids. The Lung Chi descends and helps the Large Intestine in the effort of defecation. If Lung Chi is weak or not enough, it does not give enough Chi to the Large Intestine for the act of defecation, resulting in constipation. Disorder of the Large Intestine results in abdominal pain, intestinal rumbling, diarrhea, or constipation. From the mental aspect, if deficient, one holds on to the past.

The Gall Bladder *(Dan)*

The Gall Bladder is considered a special organ among the Yang Bowels because it does not deal with food, drink, and their waste products, but stores and excretes bile, which is a refined product. The Gall Bladder sends bile downward, where it pours into the Small Intestine and helps the digestive process. The Liver and the Gall Bladder are very dependent on each other. Any disharmony of the Liver's flowing and spreading activity will affect the Gall Bladder's bile excretion. Disorder of the Gall Bladder will affect the Liver, possibly resulting in such symptoms as vomiting bitter fluids and jaundice, generated by too much bile. From the mental aspect, the Gall Bladder rules decisions according to the *Nei Jing.* The behavior characterized by anger and rash decisions may be due to excess of Gall Bladder Chi. Indecision and timidity may be a sign of Gall Bladder deficiency and weakness.

The Bladder *(Pang Guang)*

The Bladder's two major functions are receiving and excreting urine. The urine is produced by the Kidneys from the final separation of the impure fluids transmitted from the Lungs, Small Intestine, and Large Intestine. The Bladder and Kidneys have complementary functions. On the one hand, the Bladder derives the Chi necessary for the fluids' transformation from the Kidneys. On the other hand, the Kidneys depend on the Bladder to move and excrete some of their impure fluids. Symptoms of Bladder deficiency are similar to that of the Gate of Life of the Kidneys, that is, abundant, clear-colored urination. From the mental aspect, imbalance in the Bladder can fuel negative emotions such as jealousy, suspicion, and the holding of long-standing grudges.

Triple Burner (San Jiao)

There are three Burners. They are the Upper Burner, Middle Burner, and the Lower Burner. According to TCM, these are "organs" that have names but no shapes. The Upper Burner distributes fluids all over the body by the Lungs in the form of "mist." The Middle Burner, the "bubbling cauldron," digests and transports food and drink (rotting and ripening), and transports the nourishment extracted from food to all parts of the body. It also helps the Spleen to send the pure fluids up to the Upper *Jiao* and help the Stomach to direct the impure fluids downward. The Lower Burner, "the swamp," separates the essences of the food into clean and impure parts, with the excretion of the impure part.

Disorder of the Triple Burner will affect various types of Chi and Fluids in the three stages: the Upper Burner will manifest as a blockage of the Protective Chi (Lungs-dispersing function); the Middle Burner will manifest as a blockage of Nourishing Chi (Spleen-transporting function); and the blockage of Body Fluids will manifest in the Lower Burner (Bladder function of Chi transformation). These situations will result in sneezing, abdominal distention, and retention of urine respectively.

The Six Extraordinary, Curious, Or Miscellaneous Organs

These Six Extraordinary Organs function like the Yin Organs (as in storing Yin Essence and not excreting), but have the hollow shape of Yang Organs. They are: Uterus, Brain, Bones, Marrow, Gall Bladder, and Blood Vessels.

Uterus

Among the Six Extraordinary Yang Organs, the Uterus is most important because it has the function of regulating menstruation (Blood), conception, and pregnancy in women. Both the Conception (*Ren-mai*) and Governing (*Du-mai*) Vessels originate from the Kidneys but flow through the Uterus. In men, it is the *Dan Tian,* also known as "Room of Essence," that stores and produces sperm, and is directly related to the Kidneys and the Governing Vessel. If the Kidneys and the Governing Vessel are empty, it may cause disorders like impotence, premature ejaculation, clear and watery sperm, nocturnal emissions, and spermatorrhoea.

The Brain

The Brain is sometimes called the "Sea of Marrow." As in Western anatomy and physiology, the Brain controls memory, concentration, sight, hearing, touch, and smell. The Brain is closely related to the Marrow.

Marrow

In TCM the Marrow is produced by the Kidney-Essence. The marrow fills the Brain and spinal cord and forms Bone Marrow. Since it is closely related to the Kidneys, if the Kidneys are deficient, Marrow will be deficient too.

The Bones

Like all other Curious Organs, they relate to the Kidneys. They are considered Yang Organs because they store Bone Marrow. If Kidney-Essence and Marrow are deficient, the undernourished Bones will not be able to sustain the body, and there will be an inability to walk and stand.

The Blood Vessels

They are one of the six Curious Yang Organs because they contain the Blood. Again they are related to the Kidneys because Kidneys-Essence produces Marrow that contributes to producing Blood.

The Gall Bladder

It is an extraordinary Organ because it stores a pure substance called bile that is involved in breaking down impure food.

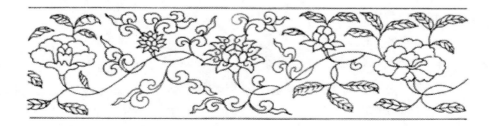

五 行

~ Chapter 6 ~

The Five-Element Theory

In the West, the universe is believed to be composed of four elements: fire, water, air, and earth. In ancient China, the constantly moving fields of forces were called the Elements. The Chinese thought more in analogies, and their logical processes were more influenced by intuitive insights and holistic thinking. In TCM the Five-Element theory describes the various stages of a natural cycle. These elements are phases of being through which things tend to move; they provide the connection between the *Zang Fu* organs and the body, and the relationship between the body and nature. It is believed that all phenomena in the universe correspond to one of five materials: wood, fire, earth, metal, and water, and that these elements are in a state of constant motion and change as they interact with one another. Each of the *Zang Fu* organs can be connected to one of the five elements.

-The Liver in its role as the regulator of Chi is thought to have similar properties to wood.
-The Lungs are felt to have clearing or cleansing properties, which are associated with the clearing or astringent properties of metal.
-The Kidneys, which serve as the regulator of metabolism, controller of water, and storehouse of essence are connected with the element of water.
-The Heart is believed to have a warming action and thus is connected to the element of fire.
-The Spleen's role in the body is one of transformation and thus is connected with the earth.

Fig. 6a. Relationships between the 5-Elements and the Organ System

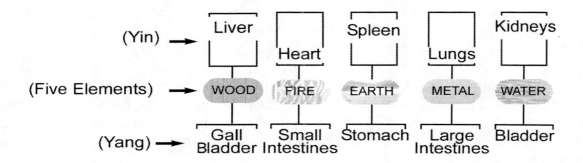

It is important to understand that the Western term "element" does not have the same meaning as the Chinese term. The Chinese see an element not as a material substance but rather as a power—a specific quality of the universe—related to laws and principles. There are emotions and feelings associated with the force of each element that express a balance or imbalance. By readjusting the relationship between the organs, balance and good health are restored.

Fig. 6b. The 5-Element Cycle

Fig. 6c. Relationships between the 5-Elements and the Organs

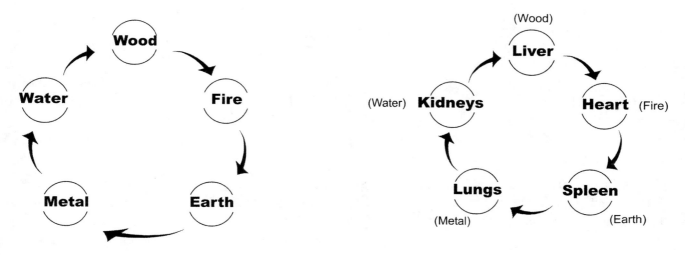

There are many different sets of corresponding relationships. The traditional method of learning about the Five Elements is to follow the seasons of the year, which are, of course, a cycle in itself.

The Element of Wood

Wood energy corresponds to the season of spring as a time of birth and is Yang. The key to understanding this element is the tree. The tree is rooted in the earth, often as deeply as its branches reach high into the sky. Through its roots, the tree takes in water and minerals for its nourishment. Its branches reach out in all directions. The tree has always symbolized growth: above and below, to the east and to the west, to the north and to the south. It has been a symbol of expansive energy. In fall and in winter, it draws back into itself and gathers strength for a new spring and summer, for a new growth ring. Liver (Yin) and Gall Bladder (Yang) are Wood organs.

The Liver embodies the power of imagination, the creative energy in us that results in growth. The Gall Bladder embodies our ability to make decisions and to assert our needs in the outer world. The Liver can be seen as the architect who designs the house while the Gall Bladder is the builder who makes decisions and arrangements so the design becomes a reality.

In the Five Elements, anger and aggression are seen in a positive light, as emotions that help us to overcome impediments to our growth. Anger and aggression are expressions of a healthy Wood element. If there is an obstacle to our growth—if we cannot find the space for expression—we feel frustrated and become angry. Anger and aggression are signs that our life energy is blocked, either from within or from without, whereas irritability, hatred, rage, and fury are perceived as signs of an imbalance in Wood. Rage is anger that has lost its purpose and gone out of control. Fury and rage typically lead to destructive behavior.

New Yang:	Birth. The energy that has been stored explodes outward, initiating a new cycle of life and activity.
Spring:	Wood energy is Yang. It rises and expands. Birth.
Human Level:	When Wood energy is abundant, we develop, we create, and we procreate. Wood strengthens the muscles, tendons, and sinews.
Organs:	Liver (Yin)—generally in charge of planning and Gall Bladder (Yang)—makes and carries out the decisions.
Color:	Green (sprouting bud).
Taste:	Sour.
Smell:	Rancid.
Direction:	East.
Sense Organ:	Eyes.
Climate:	Wind.
Sounds:	Shouting/Sighing.
Emotions:	Anger/Depression.
Tissue:	Tendons, Ligaments, and Muscles.
Function:	Keeps Chi flowing.
Imbalance:	Excess results in feeling of frustration, irritability, anger, jealousy, hatred, and rage. When depleted, there will be lethargy and depression.
To nurture:	Free expression and satisfying creativity, in harmony with natural laws and guided by *Shen*.

The Element Fire

Fire is the only element that is embodied in four organs: in the Heart, the Small Intestine, the Pericardium, or Heart Governor, and the Triple Burner. Fire governs the blood vessels: the capillaries, arteries, and veins. Its bodily fluid is perspiration.

The power of Fire is directed vertically upward, from deep in the earth up into the sky, from the material to the spiritual, from unawareness to consciousness - in the opposite direction of gravity. On the mental-emotional level, Fire brings out joy, dancing, laughter, awareness, and the ability to have an encompassing view of things. Its colors are scarlet and red.

The first Yin organ of Fire is the Heart. It is seen as the center of consciousness, feelings, and thoughts. The second Yin organ of Fire is the Pericardium, also called the Heart Cover or Heart Governor. It brings about the ability to be generous to oneself and to others, to radiate warmth, and to love. The Heart Governor expresses itself in the ability to give and in the ability to accept complaints, lamentations, criticism, and love from others.

The Chinese teachings speak of the *San Jiao* as the "three burning cavities" in the body: the chest (for breathing), the abdomen (for digestion), and the pelvis (for excretion and reproduction). The task of the Triple Burner is to coordinate these three areas of the body. The Triple Burner is the most complex of the organs, and because of this it is also the easiest to get out of balance.

Full Yang:	Growing. High level of expressive activity. Energy is highly mobile and is expended freely in all directions.
Summer:	Life flourishes (unless the heat becomes too extreme).
Human Level:	Life gently grows to its fullness with warm, all-embracing love and compassion. One has the urge to care, to give, to embrace, and to share. When Fire is given the

freedom to express itself, life is joyous, loving and peaceful, and is supported by courage, power, and wisdom. When the Fire element is in proper harmony with Nature and oneself, life has contentment, enduring vigor, a cooperative approach to life, clarity of understanding, and a freely-giving spirit.

Blocked energy: Results in "false fire"-tension, which expresses itself especially in the neck, shoulders, and head. One has the tendency to over-react and to over-extend. Physical and emotional symptoms are hysteria, insomnia, hypertension, heart attacks, strokes, and nightmares.

Organs: Heart (Yin), Small Intestine (Yang), Pericardium, and Triple Burners (to warm something up).

Color: Red.

Taste: Bitter.

Smell: Scorched.

Direction: South.

Sense Organ: Tongue.

Climate: Heat.

Sound: Laughing.

Emotions: Sadness/Joy/Happiness

Tissue: Blood and Blood Vessels.

Function: Houses the *Shen.*

Deficiency: One becomes suspicious, paranoid, loses memory.

To nurture: Feelings of compassion, love, and joy without becoming overtly excited, and the giving of ourselves.

The Element Metal

Metal symbolizes concentrated energy, an essence that keeps the universe together. Vortexes, or areas of concentrated unseen and powerful energy in nature, were used by ancient cultures for ritual purposes. These power spots and the network of energy lines on the surface of the earth are ascribed to the Metal element. The Yin organ of Metal is the lungs, the Yang organ is the Large Intestine. The Lungs receive the life energy, and the Large Intestine is the eliminator of waste. The two basic functions of the element Metal can be seen: receiving and releasing the basic forms of energy transfer with our environment. The element Metal represents our relationship to the universe—our connection to heaven and the complementary abilities of receiving and excreting, or letting go in respect to mental and physical health. The tissue that corresponds to Metal is the skin. The skin is an important eliminatory and breathing organ; plus, we are in touch with our environment through our skin. The sensory organ of Metal is the nose.

Lesser Yin: Decline. Fall energy is to be drawn inward. The vital work of the cyclic process is concluded in the Fire stage, and the outcome generated by the work is ready for gathering, processing, and storage at the Metal phase. The saying goes: "Metal keeps what is inside inside, what is outside outside; metal creates boundary."

Fall: Two processes occur in the Metal phase:
"Harvesting"- of essential product generated during the Fire phase.
"Eliminating"- of waste material also generated by the process.

Human Level:	Metal is the energy of letting go, freeing ourselves of old selves, external attachments, and emotional (in some instances, physical) entanglements.
	Metal has the ability to take in what our body needs and remove what the body does not need. Metal manifests as the state of eradication.
	In *Chinese Tonic Herbs*, Chapter One says: "The holding of strong attachments that are no longer physically present can cause (continue) intense chest and upper-back tension and pain, breathing difficulties, low resistance to colds and flu, and dull skin. Excessive letting-go can result in continuous sobbing and draining of the body's essential energy."
Organs:	Lungs (Yin), Large Intestine (Yang).
Color:	White.
Taste:	Pungent or spicy.
Smell:	Rotten.
Direction:	West.
Sense Organ:	Nose.
Climate:	Dryness.
Sound:	Crying.
Emotions:	Grief and Letting Go.
Tissue:	Skin and Body Hair.
Function:	Protection, resistance, and making things happen.
	Metal absorbs energy from the air.
Imbalance:	If not enough energy is accumulated in this phase, the *Water* phase will be unsuccessful in developing or will be depleted of energy and the entire process will cease, releasing whatever elements and energies it still has back to nature.
	If not eliminating properly, the stored energy will be weakened; then not enough energy will be left to initiate and sustain a powerful new cycle, and the ensuing *Wood* phase may flop, or otherwise generate a very weak new cycle prone to danger and potential failure. If enough energy is recaptured and stored, the process will proceed to the *Water* stage, where the energy is stored until a new round of the cycle can proceed.
To nurture:	To be able to extract the "essence" from every situation without becoming attached to the situation itself is the key to wisdom.

The Element of Water

Water is known as the cold darkness. The direction of the Water element is north. Its color is black; its time is night. Its feeling is fear. The Yin organ of Water is the Kidneys; its Yang organ is the Bladder; and its tissue is the bones. The direction of water is sinking below; its energy is a vertical flow to the center of the earth. While the energy of Fire is directed above, toward the sky, Water pulls us into the depths. It acts on the physical body like the force of gravity and leads the soul and life back to their origin, to a deep consciousness, to the central core.

The force of Water, like the energy of the other elements, affects every tissue and every cell. The force of water is present in various forms in the organism. Water is a flowing building block of the body; it constitutes 65% of the body weight and acts as a solvent and a lubricant. The constant purification of the organism through water is made possible by the Kidneys and is one of its most important functions. The flow of water through the body has nothing to do with nourishment; that is the job of the Stomach and Pancreas. Water also does not provide the body with life energy; the Lungs take care of that job.

Water flows without color and without form. Throughout the body, it picks up waste products, prevents stagnation, and makes movement, freshness, and "fluidity" of the body possible. There is no bodily function nor life process that can be carried out without water. The taste assigned to Water is salty. Salt regulates the amount of water retained by the body. The physiological mixture of the various salts in the blood and in the tissue fluids is similar to the composition of seawater. The Kidneys ensure the maintenance of the inner environment, the basis of life. Because the Kidneys are responsible for maintaining the right balance of ions in the blood and thus in the whole body, there is a close connection between the functioning of the Kidneys and the nervous system. This might be why the Chinese assigned the brain and spinal cord to the Water element.

This element represents a state of extreme Yin or death. It is a period of intense rest and a stage when energy is concentrated, awaiting a chance to explode outward to start a new phase of activity or a new cycle.

Season:	In Winter the nature energy is drawn in. Living beings safeguard their life-giving energy throughout the winter months by being less active.
	This energy is very intense and powerful.
Human Level:	In *Chinese Tonic Herbs*, Chapter One says: "Water is attracted deep within and draws with it the blood and warmth, leaving the outer-being cool (though not cold) and still (though not frozen). It produces inner heat and strength. It is our emergency reserve. (Therefore, it stores.) It regulates the water and mineral balances in the human body. It strengthens the bones (maximum Yin) and nourishes the marrow. It provides strength of the spine and ultimately determines our life span."
Organs:	Kidneys (Yin) and Urinary Bladder (Yang).
Colors:	Black and Blue.
Taste:	Salty.
Smell:	Putrid.
Direction:	North.
Sense Organ:	Ears (hearing and balancing).
Climate:	Cold.
Sounds:	Groaning/Screaming (from great fear).
Emotion:	Fear.
Tissue:	Bones and Head Hair.
Function:	Stores and conserves energy.
Deficiency:	Leads to fear, mistrust, poor resistance, a cold body, sexual difficulty, lower-back and knee pain, premature senility, and over-all bodily and mental weakness. Shortening of life span. ALL stresses drain the body-mind of Water energy.
To nurture:	Keep a balanced lifestyle. Like Metal, Water should not hold fast to things that change. One should focus on the inner self, which is permanent (Tao).

The Element of Earth

In the middle is the direction assigned to Earth; it is neither Yin nor Yang; the direction of its energy is horizontal, a closed circle. The transition periods between the seasons are also assigned to the element Earth. These are moments for looking inside and collecting oneself before a new phase begins. The elemental spirit of Earth is called *Yi*. Its homes are the Spleen and Pancreas, the Yin organs of Earth. On the physical level, the Spleen consists of two main systems, or "organs," in the body: the exocrinic part of the pancreas and the network of reticular connective tissue and endothelium that forms various anatomical structures in the body.

The main function of the Earth organs is nourishment and maintenance of the body. In the Chinese tradition, the duodenum and the first six inches of the Small Intestine are considered part of the Stomach. This is important because a large part of the absorption of nutrients takes place in the first six inches of the Small Intestine. Consequently, one can understand why the Chinese attribute the digestion of food and nourishment of the body to the Earth organs and, only to a lesser extent, to the Small Intestine. However, "nourishment" refers not only to providing nutrients but also to providing oxygen via the red blood cells to every cell in the body. The red blood cells are formed in the red bone marrow that belongs to the Spleen. Another aspect of maintaining the body's integrity is the work of the immune system, whose components belong to the Spleen. The red bone marrow generates the B-lymphocytes, which produce antibodies; the lymphatic organs (primarily the lymph glands and the Spleen) generate the T-lymphocytes, which are programmed to fight specific antigens. The Spleen is the mother organ of the physical body and also the organ responsible for fertility, pregnancy, and birth. The Spleen regulates the distribution of water and blood. The organ tissues that are assigned to Earth are the connective tissue, fat tissue, and muscle fibers. The Spleen's Yang organ is the Stomach, and its sensory organ the mouth.

Maturation:	It represents the center, the balance, and the harmony of all the other elemental energies. Earth is always present and dominant in all elemental energies. Passive energy.
Season:	Indian Summer (between two seasons)—late September and early October.
Human Level:	Homeostasis, and the balance of life that assures our continuation.
Organs:	Spleen (Yin). Gives energy to the process of digestion. Stomach (Yang) executes digestion.
Color:	Yellow.
Taste:	Sweet.
Smell:	Fragrant.
Direction:	Center.
Sense Organ:	Mouth.
Climate:	Dampness (which can destroy Spleen. Stomach suffers from not enough moisture—digestion problems).
Sound:	Singing.
Emotion:	Pensiveness.
Tissue:	Flesh (between skin and muscle—body fat).
Function:	Digestion (food and ideas).
Excess:	An individual becomes worried and becomes obsessed with details, losing perspective of the big picture, which results in "tunnel vision," hypochondria, digestive and blood disorders, and, in women, menstrual disorders.
Deficiency:	The mind becomes cloudy while the body becomes heavy and lethargic, often waterlogged with fatigue and resultant depression, forgetfulness.
To nurture:	Always seeing life from a wide perspective while remaining physically and emotionally centered.

The Four Cycles

The *Sheng* Cycle: This cycle describes the transition from one element to the next, from one phase to the next. Wood transforms into Fire, Fire into Earth, Earth into Metal, Metal into Water, and Water back into Wood. In Chinese texts, the changes are shown in the following way: you use wood to make fire; when the fire has burned, it becomes ashes, it becomes earth; in the depths of earth, metals and minerals are compressed and created; water condenses on metal; or from heaven, the kingdom of metal, comes the rain; water nourishes the plants so they can grow; hence, water creates wood; when a lot of wood is piled up, then the fire will burn brighter and longer; the burning of fields creates new, fertile earth. The manifestation of energy of every element in the cycle is dependent upon the nourishment it gets from the element before it in the cycle; therefore, this cycle is also called The Cycle of Nourishment.

For the observed processes in nature and the cosmos, the characteristics of the individual elements play less of a role than their actual interplay. In every life process, the elements balance one another, create one another, and block one another. The four laws governing the relationship of the elements to one another are: the Cycle of Creation (*Sheng*—the law of mother and child), the Cycle of Checking-Up and Control (*Ko*—the grandmother controls the grandchild), the Cycle of Rebellion (grandchild against grandmother), and the Cycle of Withdrawal (greedy child who sucks the mother dry). These four cycles describe the phases of growth and the physiological interplay of the organs and show how the elements are connected to one another, and how everything that happens has an effect on everything else. The *Sheng* cycle portrays a closed circle. If the circle is broken at any point and one element is unable to nourish the next, the result is "malnourishment." The Chinese call this, relative to the previous element, the "child." The nourishing element is the "mother." The child of one element is the mother of the next.

The cycle of creation and building has, as its natural polarity, breakdown and destruction of outlived structures. Just as every element has a mother who nourishes it, every element also has a grandmother who is responsible for its upbringing and its proper growth.

In the *Ko* cycle the law is portrayed as: water puts out fire; fire melts metal; metal (in the form of a saw or ax) cuts wood; wood (as a plant or tree) breaks through the surface of the earth; earth dams up the path of water.

Fig. 6d. Five-Element Interrelationships

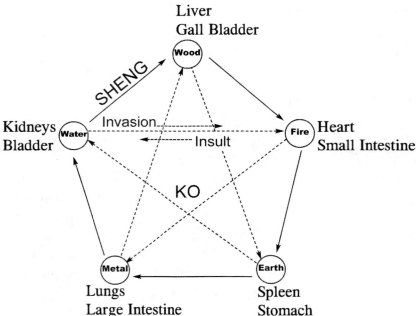

54

The success of Traditional Chinese Medicine in treating chronic illnesses is, for the most part, based on restoring the balance of the elements. In many cases, this is possible via knowledge of the four cycles and help from suitable therapeutic methods: diet, herbs, breathing and physical exercises like Chi Gong and Tai Chi, meridian massage, Shiatsu, acupressure, acupuncture, and meditation.

The Main Corresponding Relationships of the Five Elements

	WOOD	FIRE	EARTH	METAL	WATER
SEASONS	Spring	Summer	In. Summer	Fall	Winter
DIRECTIONS	East	South	Center	West	North
COLORS	Green	Red	Yellow	White	Black
TASTES	Sour	Bitter	Sweet	Pungent/ Spicy	Salty
SMELLS	Rancid	Scorched	Fragrant	Rotten	Putrid
CLIMATES	Wind	Heat	Dampness	Dryness	Cold
STAGES OF DEVELOPMENT	Birth/ Expansion	Growth/ Combustion	Maturation/ Transformation	Decline/ Contraction	Death/ Consolidation
YIN AND YANG	New (Lesser) Yang	Full Yang	Center	Lesser Yin	Full Yin
YIN ORGANS	Liver	Heart/P.C.	Spleen	Lungs	Kidneys
YANG BOWELS	Gall Bladder	Small Int./ T.B.	Stomach	Large Int.	Bladder
TISSUES	Tendons/ Ligaments/ Muscles	Blood/ Blood Vessels	Flesh	Skin/ Body Hair	Bones/ Head Hair
EMOTIONS	Anger/ Depression	Joy/Sadness	Pensiveness	Grief	Fear
SOUNDS	Shouting	Laughing	Singing	Crying	Groaning
SENSE ORGANS	Eyes	Tongue	Mouth	Nose	Ears
FUNCTIONS	Keeps Chi flowing	Houses the *Shen*	Digestion	Protects	Stores
PHYSIOLOGICAL SYSTEMS	Neuro-muscular	Cardio-vascular	Gastro-intestinal	Respiratory	Central Nervous

~Chapter 7~

Meridians and Acupuncture Points

In TCM every part of the body is connected by the network of energy. The physical part of the body is a manifestation of the energy part of the body. Meridians are the channels that Chi and sometimes blood flow through, and the acupressure and acupuncture points are the places where the flow of Chi can be tapped into. Meridians are a network connecting the interior with the exterior—the internal organs with the surface of the body, tissue with spirit. The meridian system consists mainly of the Twelve Organ Meridians (also called the Twelve Regular Channels). Each of these pertains to and connects with a particular *Zang* or *Fu* organ (see Chapter 5, page 39 for explanation); the organ meridian is the main energy channel that connects the particular organ with other organs and the surface of the body.

The function of the meridians is to provide for the circulation of Chi throughout the body, thus nourishing the tissues and linking up the whole body so as to keep the internal organs, four limbs, muscles, tendons, and bones intact and functioning as one unit. Each Internal Organ has an energetic extension from the Organ to the surface of the body. Since the Chinese Medical system looks at the human body as a whole, all organs work together to create a whole person.

Like the Internal Organs system, the meridian system also has a pairing system. The Twelve Organ Meridians form six pairs. Each Yin meridian is assigned to a Yang meridian of the *same* element. These pairs are also called Coupled Meridians. Each *Zang* organ is paired with a *Fu* organ of the same element. Their physiological, emotional, intellectual, and spiritual functions are closely related; each *Zang* organ embodies the Yin power, each *Fu* the Yang force of the corresponding element. The Twelve Regular Channels are:

Yin	Yang
Heart	Small Intestine
Liver	Gall Bladder
Lungs	Large Intestine
Kidneys	Bladder
Spleen	Stomach
Pericardium	Triple Burner (Warmer)

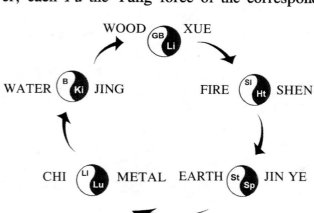

Fig. 7A. Interrelationships between 5-Elements, Organs, and Body Essences

The reasons for the pairing of these particular meridians are:

1. The two meridians of each pair are connected at the extremities, via the entry and exit points. For example, the Lung and Large Intestine meridians are connected at the thumb and first finger, where the Lung meridian ends and the Large Intestine meridian begins.
2. In the Body Clock, one partner follows the other.

Fig. 7B. Chinese Meridian Body Clock

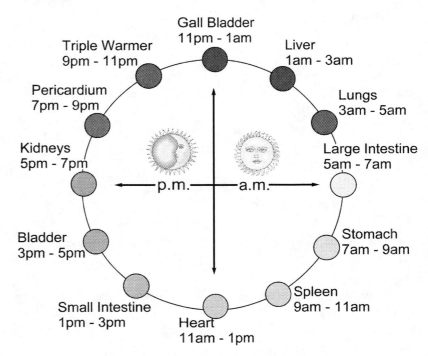

3. Each meridian has a *Connecting meridian* that links it to its partner.
4. Each meridian also has a *Divergent meridian* that connects it with the Internal Organ associated with its partner.
5. Each pair is associated with one of the Five Elements, so the same Five-Element associations (season, color, etc.) apply to both meridians.
6. The paired Organs' meridians usually share functions. For example, the Large Intestine and the Lungs are both eliminative Organs: the Large Intestine eliminates digestive waste, and the Lungs release carbon dioxide and other gaseous wastes.

From this pairing we can trace back and connect with all the other theories that we have studied thus far.

Four Segments of the Channels

There are four segments of the Channels. All Channels begin at the *Organs* themselves. Then the second segment is the *Interior Branch*. Here the Chi runs within a pathway of the body, and usually this branch is too deep to be affected by the acupuncture needles. The third segment is the *Exterior Branch* where all the acupuncture points are located. The fourth segment (the *Antique Points*) actually is part of the third segment but is located at the end of each Channel.

Fig. 7C. Four Segments of Channels

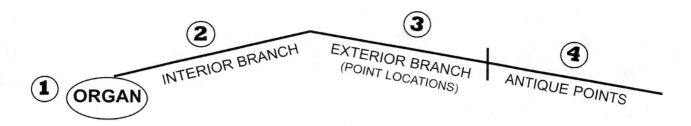

Eleven Important Considerations in the Study of the Meridians

1. All the Points have distal and local effects.
2. All 12 Channels are bilateral.
3. All Yang Channels begin or end at the Head.
4. All Yin Channels begin or end at the Chest.
5. All Yang Channels descend.
6. All Yin Channels ascend.
7. The traditional Chinese anatomical position is with the arms raised.
8. The more distal the Points are, the stronger the Chi, therefore affecting the related Organ the greatest.
9. The Points at the extremities have a deeper effect on the Organs themselves, especially the Antique Points.
10. From the point of view of Yin and Yang, the Organs and Interior Branch are Yin.
11. The Exterior Branch and the Antique Points are Yang.

In order to remember the concept of descending and ascending of the Channels, we can think of the three Powers. Heaven shines down the Chi to humans while the Earth grows plants upward to Heaven.

The Anatomical Arrangement of the Meridians

One meridian of each pair is Yin and one is Yang. The Yin meridians flow up the body, and the Yang meridians flow down.

1. All the leg Yin meridians begin at the feet and flow up to the Chest (K, Sp, Li).
2. All the leg Yang meridians begin on the head and flow down to the toes (B, GB, St).
3. All the arm Yin meridians begin on the upper chest and flow down to the fingers (H, P, Lu).
4. All the arm Yang meridians begin at the fingers and flow up the arm and up the neck to the end on the head (LI, SI, TB).

The Yin meridians are, in general, located on the inside, soft surfaces of the body (the inside of the arms and legs, the front of the body). The Yang meridians are usually located on the outer, firmer, bonier surfaces of the body (the back, the sides of the body, the head, the outside of the arms and legs).

There are 6 Yin Channels and 6 Yang Channels. Out of that there are 3 Yin Arm Channels and 3 Yang Arm Channels, 3 Yin Leg Channels and 3 Yang Leg Channels. Each pair of Channels of the upper body communicates with one pair of the lower body's Channels. That is called the Arm/Leg Channel communication.

There are 6 energetic layers of Channel communication: *Tai Yang*, *Shao Yang*, *Yang Ming* (beginning of Yang), *Tai Yin*, *Jue Yin*, and *Shao Yin* (most Yin part of Body).

The 3 Yin Channels of the Arm are:	*Tai Yin* – Lungs (Lu)
	Jue Yin – Pericardium (P)
	Shao Yin – Heart (H)
The 3 Yang Channels of the Arm are:	*Tai Yang* – Small Intestine (SI)
	Shao Yang – San Jiao/Triple Burner (TB)
	Yang Ming – Large Intestine (LI)
The 3 Yin Channels of the Leg are:	*Tai Yin* – Spleen (Sp)
	Jue Yin – Liver (Li)
	Shao Yin – Kidneys (K)
The 3 Yang Channels of the Leg are:	*Tai Yang* – Bladder (B)
	Shao Yang – Gall Bladder (GB)
	Yang Ming – Stomach (St)

These are represented as:

Arm/Hand Channels (More Yang)	Energetic Layers	Leg/Foot Channels (More Yin)
SI	*Tai Yang*	B
TB	*Shao Yang*	GB
LI	*Yang Ming*	St
Lu	*Tai Yin*	Sp
P	*Jue Yin*	Li
H	*Shao Yin*	K
(FIRE)		(WATER)

A Chinese medical doctor can diagnose a patient by using this chart. Sometimes a weakened Organ will pull energy from across a Channel energy layer from another Organ (e.g., Lungs pull Spleen).

Extra Channels

The two extra Channels are the Governing Vessel and the Conception Vessel. They are the most important channels in the body, because the Governing Vessel governs all the 6 primary Yang Channels and the Conception Vessel governs all the 6 primary Yin Channels. Both are Yin and Yang polarities of the *Yuan Chi*. (See Chapter 3, page 21 for an explanation.) They regulate the functions of the entire endocrine system.

Special Points

All Well *(Jing)* Points are acupuncture points at the tips of the fingers or the toes where the meridians begin or end. The Well Points are also called the *Tendino-Muscular* Points (Channels). The *Wei Chi,* as explained in Chapter 3, circulates at these points. Other than that, *Ying Chi,* as discussed in Chapter 3, circulates in all the 12 primary meridians. Other special points like Source Points, Lo Points, Alarm Points, Yu Points, Entry Points, and Exit Points will be discussed below.

Source Points

The Source Points are the "balancing points" in that they reestablish the energy balance of the meridian by either sedating or tonifying the meridian based on the need of the body. The Source Points are located both in the hands and feet and ankles and wrists, and are located on the meridian that they control. A point can be manipulated in a clockwise direction to tonify or counter-clockwise direction to sedate the meridian. The Source Points are: Lu 9, H 7, P 7, St 42, Li 3, TB 4, SI 4, LI 4, Sp 3, K 3, B 64, & GB 40.

Lo Points

Page 39 of the *Intermediate & Advanced Acupressure Course Booklet* states: "Between each meridian pair, there is a connective meridian, which serves to balance the relationship between the two meridians by allowing energy to flow between them. The connective meridian runs between the Lo Points." When there is an energy imbalance between two meridians of a pair, Lo Points, or Connecting Points are stimulated in order to balance their relationship. The Lo Point can also be used to tonify or sedate depending if there is an excess or deficiency, or to balance the energy on the left and right halves of the same meridian. The Lo Points are P 6, Lu 7, H 5, St 40, Li 5, GB 37, SI 7, LI 6, TB 5, Li 5, Sp 4, K 4, St 40, B 58, & GV 37.

Alarm Points

The Alarm Points are used to diagnose the condition of the 12 primary organs. Therefore, tenderness on the Alarm Points indicates an imbalance in the associated organ. Alarm Points are located on the chest and abdomen. The front of the body is considered a Yin surface, and these points are usually associated with Yin conditions and become sensitive when there is an imbalance in the associated organ. Alarm Points are traditionally considered tonification points. Alarm Points include: St 25 (LI), CV 14 (H), Lu 1 (Lung), CV 17 (P), Li 14 (Li), GB 24 (GB), CV 12 (St), CV 5 (TB), CV 4 (SI), CV 3 (B), GB 25 (K), Li 14 (Li), GV 24 (GB), Li 13 (Sp), & GV 25 (K).

Yu Points

Yu Points can directly stimulate the internal organs via the spinal nerves. They are located on the back along the inner bladder meridian and can tonify either the Yang or the Yin. The Governing Vessel Points nearest the sensitive Yu Point can also be used. Going down the right side of the spine, the Yu Points include: B 13 Lung, B 14 Pericardium, B 15 Heart, B 18 Liver, B 19 Gall Bladder, B 20 Spleen, B 21 Stomach, B 22 Triple Burner, B 23 Kidney, B 25 Large Intestine, B 27 Small Intestine, and B 28 Bladder. On the left side of the spine, starting near the shoulder blade and going down to the sacrum, the Yu Points are: B 38, B 42, B 47, & B 48.

"Yu Mansion" (K 27) is considered the master point for all the Yu Points. K 27 is located bilaterally under the clavicle where it joins the rib cage. Hold the master Yu Point with any Yu Point to help the Yu Point release.

Entry & Exit Points

The Entry and Exit Points are the points where energy is passed from one meridian to the next, for instance, from the Lung to Large Intestine to the Stomach meridians, etc. Often, but not always, these points are the first and last points on a meridian. The Entry and Exit Points are used to tonify and sedate the meridians. Therefore, in order to sedate a meridian, you can either sedate the Entry Point when the *preceding* meridian in the energy cycle as shown in the diagram below is deficient or sedate the Exit Point when the *following* meridian in the energy cycle is deficient.

The Source Points, Lo Points, Alarm Points, Yu Points, and Entry and Exit Points are included in the information on the charts for the different meridians that begin on the next page.

Cycles

The circulation of Chi in the Twelve Organ Meridians has its own sequence. It is different from the laws of the four cycles discussed in Chapter 6. Chi flows in the meridians in the following order: from Lung to Large Intestine to Stomach to Spleen to Heart to Small Intestine to Bladder to Kidney to Pericardium to Triple Burner to Gall Bladder to Liver. From the Liver meridian the circulating Chi flows back to the Lung meridian to start a new cycle. The circulation of Chi in the body is a continuous flow similar to the blood circulation.

Fig. 7D. A diagrammatic representation of Chi flow within the meridians

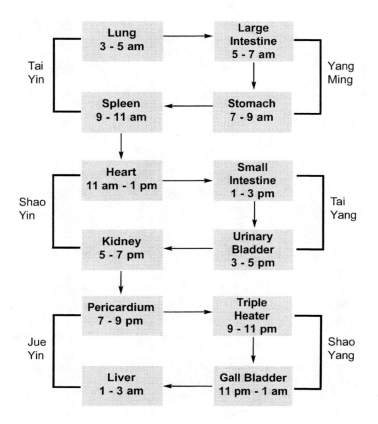

LUNG MERIDIAN

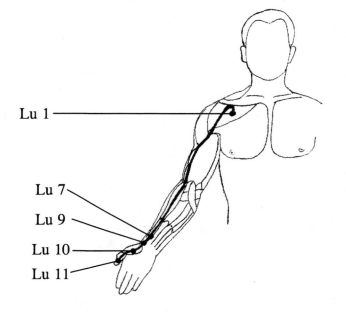

Base Points:

Lu 1

B 13

Lu 1
Lu 7
Lu 9
Lu 10
Lu 11

Source Point:
Lu 9

Yin or Yang:
Yin - Zang

Paired Meridian:
Large Intestine/Yang

5 Element:
Metal

Time Cycle:
3 A.M. - 5 A.M.

Relationships:
Constructive – K/B
Destructive – Li/GB

Important Points on the Lung Meridian*

Point		Location	Symptoms of Imbalance
Lu 1 "Middle Palace"	Entry & Alarm Pont	In the first intercostal space, 2 *cun*** lateral to the nipple	Grief, upper back & shoulder tension, arm, chest problems, breathing
Lu 7 "Narrow Defile"	Lo Point Exit Point	In the radial groove, 2 *cun* proximal to the wrist fold	Asthma, cough, stiff neck, conception vessel disorders
Lu 9 "Great Abyss"	Source Point	In the radial groove at the wrist fold	Emotions, wrist, asthma, coughing, chest pain
Lu 10 "Fish Region"	Fire Point	On the palmar surface, in the 1st metacarpal bone, at the junction of the "white & red" skin	Chest, neck & abdominal pain coughing blood, asthma
Lu 11 "Young Merchant"	Wood Point	On the radial side of the thumb at the corner of the nail	Tonsillitis, epilepsy, fever

Traditional Indication for Use of Lung Meridian

Anxiety	Bronchitis	Depression	Mucous, excessive
Arm pain/paralysis	Chest pain	Edema in the face	Pharynx
Asthma	Congestion	Insomnia	Skin problems
Breathing problems	Coughing	Lung problems	Tonsillitis & voice problems

* These Meridian charts (pp.62 - 80) are based on information from the *Intermediate & Advanced Acupressure Course Booklet* by the Acupressure Institute School of Massage Therapy, ©1984 by Michael Reed Gach.
** A Chinese system of measurement. See page 86 for more information.

LARGE INTESTINE MERIDIAN

Base Points:

LI 1

B 27-30

GB 21

B 13

B 48

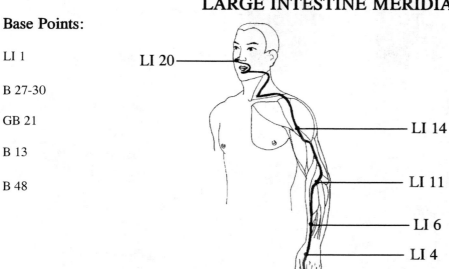

Source Point:
LI 4 (Hoku)

Yin or Yang:
Yang - Fu

Paired Meridian:
Lung /Yin

5 Element:
Metal

Time Cycle:
5 A.M. – 7 A.M.

Relationships:
Constructive – K/B
Destructive – Li/GB

Important Points on the Large Intestine Meridian

Point		Location	Symptoms of Imbalance
LI 1 "Merchant Yang"		On the index finger at the base of the nail (thumb side)	Fever, cough, swollen throat, sore throat
LI 4* "Hoku"	Source Point Entry Point	In the webbing between the thumb and index finger. Press into hollow against 2nd metacarpal of index finger.	Constipation, headache, toothache, tonsillitis, facial paralysis, shoulder/arm tension, lower jaw problems, common cold, insomnia, late menstrual period

LI 4's are two of the four gates. It is forbidden to work this area on pregnant women until labor because it opens the descending or yang meridians.

Point		Location	Symptoms of Imbalance
LI 6 "Side Passage"	Lo Point	3 *cun* above wrist on the radial side of the arm	Fever, tonsillitis, tinnitus, toothache
LI 11 "Crooked Pond"		At the external extremity of the elbow crease	Constipation, elbow, arm, & shoulder pain, upper extremity paralysis, eczema
LI 14 "Outer Arm Bone"		On the lateral surface of the arm in the deltoid V	Arm swollen, numb, or painful, stiff neck, toothache, stiff neck
LI 20 "Welcoming Perfume"	Exit Point	In the small depression at the outside lower corner of the nostril	Nasal congestion, facial paralysis, face swollen

Traditional Indication for Use of Large Intestine Meridian

Arthritis	Coughing	Nose bleeds	Hypersalivation	Tonsillitis
Boils	Diarrhea	Paralysis of arms/face	Mouth dry	Toothache
Congestion	Difficult breathing	Sense of smell weak	Shoulder pain	Throat spasms
Constipation	Headache	Sore throat	Skin problems	

STOMACH MERIDIAN

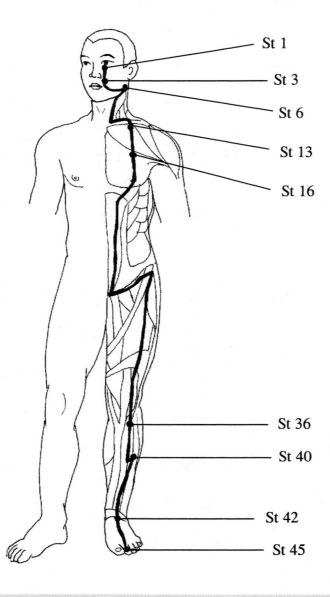

Base Points:

St 36 (3 Miles)

St 13

B 21

St 16

St 1
St 3
St 6
St 13
St 16

St 36
St 40
St 42
St 45

Source Point:
St 42

Yin or Yang:
Yang - Fu

Paired Meridian:
Spleen/Yin

5 Element:
Earth

Time Cycle:
7 A.M. – 9 A.M.

Relationships:
Constructive – Lu/LI
Destructive – K/B

Important Points on the Stomach Meridian

Point		Location	Symptoms of Imbalance
St 1 "Receive Tears"	Entry Point	Just below the center of the eye in an indentation on the bony ridge	Eye problem
St 3 "Facial Beauty"	St/LI Reunion	Just under the cheekbone, 1 *cun* from the nostril. Press up on underside of cheekbone.	Used for local conditions (headaches, sinuses, facial paralysis, jaw tension), nausea
St 6 "Jaw Chariot"	St/GB Reunion Point	Anterior and superior to the angle of the jaw at the prominence of the masseter muscle, when the jaw is shut (often sore)	Inflammation of jaw, pain, grinding teeth

Important Points on the Stomach Meridian (continued)

Point		Location	Symptoms of Imbalance
St 13 "Chi Door"		Just below the midpoint of the clavicle	Shoulder tension, chest pain and tension, asthma, bronchitis, paralysis, eczema
St 16 "Breast Window"		In the 3rd intercostal space, directly above the nipple	Cough, asthma, mastitis, heartburn, lactation, emotional distress
St 36 "Three Miles"	Sea of Nourishment	In the depression between the tibia and the tibialis anticus, 3 *cun* below the patella (knee cap)	General tonic point, stomach disorders, constipation, distal point for symptoms near stomach points on neck & head
St 40 "Abundant Splendor"	Lo Point	Midway from the head of the fibula to the lateral malleolus, between tibia and fibula	Coughing phlegm, dizziness, schizophrenia, leg problems
St 42 "Rushing Yang"	Source Point Exit Point	1.5 *cun* distal to the transverse malleolus crease, at the highest spot of the dorsum of the foot where an artery can be palpated	Toothache, gum problems, vomiting, yawning, foot problems
St 45 "General Exchange"		Lateral corner of the base of the 2nd toenail	Sinusitis, tonsillitis, swollen face, cerebral anemia, fainting

Traditional Indication for Use of Stomach Meridian

Abdominal disorders	Deafness	Fatigue	Jaw/mouth problems
Anorexia	Diarrhea	Flatulence	Leg pain, paralysis
Arthritis of leg & knee	Epilepsy	Genital problems	Obsession
Breast problems	Excessive sympathy	Headaches	Tonsillitis
Cough, emphysema	Eye problems	Hernia	Vomiting

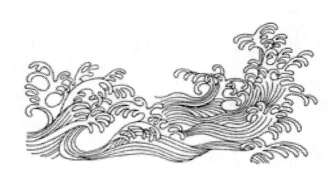

SPLEEN MERIDIAN

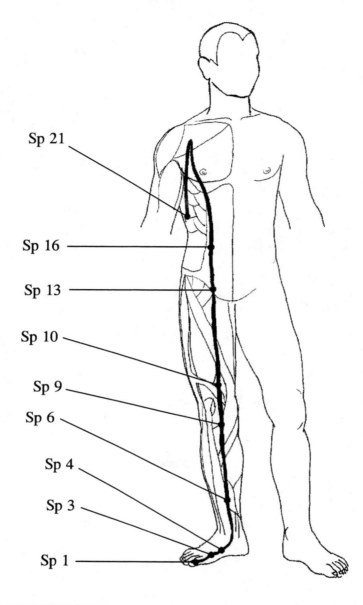

Base Points:

Sp 4

Sp 13

Sp 16

B 20

Source Point:
Sp 3

Yin or Yang:
Yin - Zang

Paired Meridian:
Stomach/Yang

5 Element:
Earth

Time Cycle:
9 A.M. – 11 A.M.

Relationships:
Constructive – Lu/LI
Destructive – K/B

Important Points on the Spleen Meridian

Point		Location	Symptoms of Imbalance
Sp 1 "Hidden White"	Entry Point	At the medial angle of the base of the big toenail	Insomnia, vomiting, irregular menstruation, hyperacidity
Sp 3 "Most White"	Source Point	At the base of the knuckle of the big toe, on the line where the dorsal and plantar surfaces meet	Constipation, diarrhea, vomiting, hernia
Sp 4 "Grandfather/ Grandson"	Lo Point	1 *cun* proximal to Sp 3	Foot cramps, stomach disorders, menstrual cramps, pain due to injury of the testicles, epilepsy

Important Points on the Spleen Meridian (continued)

Point		Location	Symptoms of Imbalance
Sp 6 "3 Yin Meeting"	Reunion of Sp,K,Li	3 *cun* above internal malleolus	Genital pain and disorders, diarrhea, nervous depression, menstrual disorders, labor
Sp 9 "Fountain of Yin"		Under the head of the tibia	Used for any yin condition, bleeding, edema, knee problems, menstrual irregularity
Sp 10 "Sea of Blood"		2 *cun* above the superior border of the patella, medial aspect of thigh-midline. Press up onto femur.	Menstrual problems, knee problems, edema
Sp 13 "Mansion Cottage"		In the groin 4 *cun* lateral to the midline of the body, just above ligament	Sexual frustration, pelvic tension, hernia, menstrual problems, indigestion, abdominal pain, not grounded, uterine hemorrhage
Sp 16 "Abdomen Sorrow"		At the junction of the 9th rib cartilage to the 8th rib, below the nipple, press up into rib.	Side ache, ulcer, hypo or hyper acidity, diaphragm tensions, hiccoughs, any abdominal dysfunction
Sp 21 "Big Wrapping"	Exit Point Grand Lo Point	On mid-auxiliary line in 7th intercostal space, 6 *cun* below armpit	Chest and side pains, general aches

Traditional Indication for Use of Spleen Meridian

Abdominal cramps/pains	Diabetes	Hemorrhage	Menstrual cramps
Anorexia	Diarrhea	Hemorrhoids	Muscle spasms
Big toe problems	Edema	Hypoglycemia	Vomiting
Constipation	Fatigue	Indigestion	Weakness in legs
Depression	Genital disorders	Insomnia	Used during labor

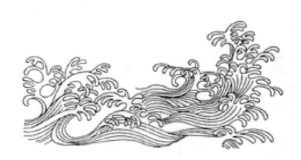

HEART MERIDIAN

Base Points:

B 38

Cv 17
(Sea of Tranquility)

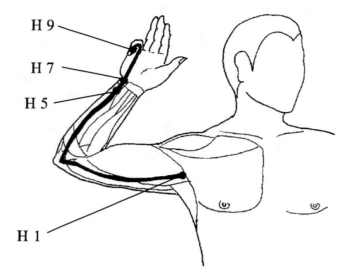

H 9

H 7

H 5

H 1

Source Point:
H 7

Yin or Yang:
Yin - Zang

Paired Meridian:
Small Intestine/Yang

5 Element:
Fire

Time Cycle:
11 A.M. – 1 P.M.

Relationships:
Constructive – Sp/St
Destructive – Lu/LI

Important Points on the Heart Meridian

Point		Location	Symptoms of Imbalance
H 1 "Extreme Spring"	Entry Point	Center of the armpit (hold gently)	Chest pain, hysteria, impulsiveness
H 5 "Penetrating Inside"	Lo Point	On the ulna side of wrist, 1 *cun* above H 7	Dizziness, vertigo, hysteria, anxiety, palpitations, fear
H 7 "Spirit Door"	Source Point	On the ulna side of the wrist, on the anterior border of the pisiform bone	Insomnia, anxiety, hysteria, stage fright, cardiac arrhythmia, hot flashes
H 9 "Lesser Rushing"	Exit Point	At the corner of the base of the nail on the inside of the little finger	Emergency heart point, palpitations, melancholy, heart attack, high fever

Traditional Indication for Use of Heart Meridian

Anxiety	Diarrhea	Headache	Melancholy, depression
Chest pain	Dry cough	Heart pain, palpitations	Menopause
Cold (especially in arms)	Extreme sweating	Hysteria	Muteness
Confusion	Extreme thirst	Insomnia	Speech disorders

SMALL INTESTINE MERIDIAN

Base Points:

SI 10

SI 14

SI 12

SI 11

SI 19
SI 14
SI 12
SI 10
SI 11
SI 7
SI 4
SI 3
SI 1

Source Point:
SI 4

Yin or Yang:
Yang - Fu

Paired Meridian:
Heart /Yin

5 Element:
Fire

Time Cycle:
1 P.M. – 3 P.M.

Relationships:
Constructive – Sp/St
Destructive – Lu/LI

Important Points on the Small Intestine Meridian

Point		Location	Symptoms of Imbalance
SI 1 "Little Marsh"	Entry Point	At the outside corner of the base of the little fingernail	Headache, eye problems, deficient lactation, confusion
SI 3 "Back-Stream"	Balances Governing Vessel	When the hand is clenched, at the deepest transverse crease of the palm	Stiff neck and back, ear problems, epilepsy, headache
SI 4 "Wrist Bone"	Source Point	Just proximal to the base of the 5th metacarpal on the ulnar edge of the hand	Shoulder tension, arthritis in elbow, wrist, and finger, ear problems, headache
SI 7 "Straight Branch"	Lo Point	At posterior margin of ulna, 5 *cun* above wrist	Stiff neck, pain or spasms in the forearm or hand, mental disorders

Important Points on the Small Intestine Meridian (continued)

Point		Location	Symptoms of Imbalance
SI 10 "Shoulder Blade Point"		Where the humerus and scapula meet, below the acromion	Upper back, shoulders, arm tension or pain
SI 11 "Heavenly Ancestor"	Arm & Scapula Point	In the center of the scapula (infrascapular fossa)	Shoulder pain, frustration
SI 12 "Facing the Wind"	Reunion of SI, LI, TB, GB	In the center of the suprascapular fossa, directly above SI 11	Shoulder numbness or aching of upper extremities
SI 14 "Shoulder Correspondence"	Shoulder Release Point	Superior to the upper inside tip of the scapula	Spasm, pain, or tightness of the shoulder and/or neck
SI 19 "Listening Palace"	Exit Point	In the depression that appears when the mouth is opened (between) the tragus and the mandible joint	Tinnitus, deafness

Traditional Indication for Use of Small Intestine Meridian

Arm pain or paralysis	Confusion	Headache	Sore throat
Arthritis in the arms, hands, or shoulders	Deafness	Puffy cheeks	Tinnitus
	Eye problems	Shoulder tension	Tonsillitis

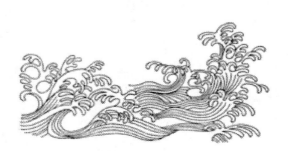

BLADDER MERIDIAN

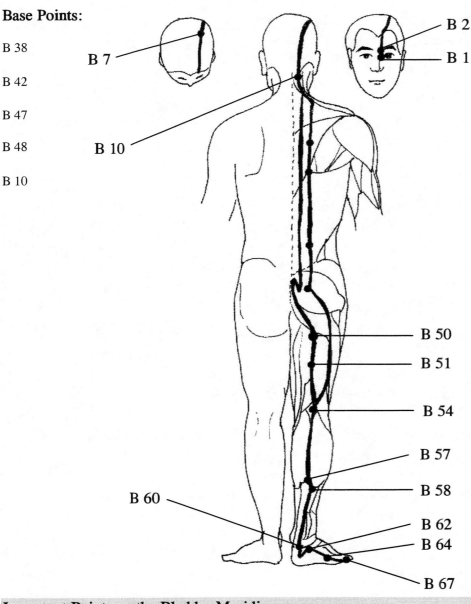

Base Points:

B 38

B 42

B 47

B 48

B 10

B 7

B 10

B 2

B 1

B 50

B 51

B 54

B 57

B 58

B 60

B 62

B 64

B 67

Source Point:
B 64

Ying or Yang:
Yang - Fu

Paired Meridian:
Kidneys/Yin

5 Element:
Water

Time Cycle:
3 P.M. – 5 P.M.

Relationships:
Constructive – Li/GB
Destructive – H/SI

Important Points on the Bladder Meridian

Point		Location	Symptoms of Imbalance
B 1 "Eyes Bright"	Entry Point	At the bottom of the hollow at the inner corner of the eye	Eyes, facial paralysis
B 2 "Collect Bamboo"	Pituitary Point	Directly above B 1 at the inside of the eyebrow	Sinuses, eyes, allergic sneezing, headache
B 7 "Penetrating Heaven"	Brain Tonic Point	1 *cun* lateral to GV 20	Headache, nose (smell), eyes

Important Points on the Bladder Meridian (continued)

Point		Location	Symptoms of Imbalance
B 10 "Heavenly Pillar"	Sea of Energy Point	Just below the base of the occipital ridge, between the 1st and 2nd vertebrae, 1 ½ *cun* from the GV	Neck tension, headache, blocked nose, sore throat
B 50 "Receive & Support"		In the center of the transverse buttock fold	Sciatica, hemorrhoids, leg paralysis
B 51 "Prosperous Gate"		6 *cun* below B 50	Back pain, thigh problems, sciatica
B 54 "Commanding Middle"		In the center of the back of the knee (popliteal fold)	Sciatica, back pain or stiffness, knee pain, headaches, stiff neck, hip disorders, arthritis
B 57 "Supporting Mountain"		Midway between B 54 and the heel, at the bottom of the calf muscle bulge	Hemorrhoids, constipation, lumbago
B 58 "Soaring"	Lo Point	At posterior margin of fibula, 1 *cun* below & lateral to B 57	Epilepsy, dizziness, lumbago
B 60 "High Mountain"		Midway between the lateral malleolus (outer ankle bone) and the Achilles tendon	Lower backache or pain, convulsions in little children
B 62 "Extended Meridian"		Directly below the tip of the external malleolus, ½ *cun* lateral to its lower border	Epilepsy, headache, dizziness, uterus spasm, backache
B 64 "Capital Bone"	Source Point	Below the tuberosity of the 5th metatarsal, where "red and white" skin meet	Headache, dizziness, leg pain, epilepsy, lumbago
B 67 "Extremity of Yin"	Exit Point	The outside corner of the base of the little toenail	Eye pain, difficult labor, malposition of fetus, dysuria, urinary dysfunctions

Traditional Indication for Use of Bladder Meridian

Back problems	Epilepsy	Hemorrhoids	Pain or spasms in calf
Cystitis, urinary problems	Eye problems	Hip pain	Paralysis
Diabetes	Genital disorders	Neck pain	Sciatica
Ear problems	Headaches	Nosebleeds	Stiff little toe

KIDNEY MERIDIAN

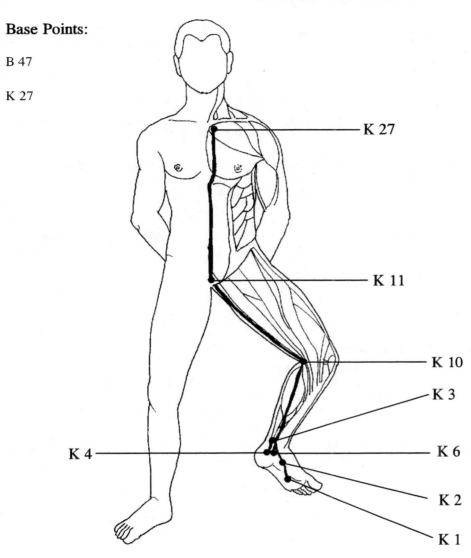

Base Points:

B 47

K 27

K 27

K 11

K 10

K 3

K 6

K 4

K 2

K 1

Source Point:
K 3

Yin or Yang:
Yin - Zang

Paired Meridian:
Bladder/Yang

5 Element:
Water

Time Cycle:
5 P.M. – 7 P.M.

Relationships:
Constructive – Li/GB
Destructive – H/SI

Important Points on the Kidney Meridian

Point		Location	Symptoms of Imbalance
K 1 "Bubbling Spring"	Entry Point	On the sole of the foot, at the base of the ball of the foot, between the two pads	Retention of urine, pent-up emotions, fainting, coma, shock, epilepsy, dry or sore throat, convulsions
K 2 "Blazing Valley"	Fire Point	On the inside of the foot, just under the navicular prominence (arch of the foot)	Cystitis, diabetes, night sweats, irregular menstruation, prolapse of uterus & other dysfunctions of the sexual organs
K 3 "Mountain Stream"	Source Point	Behind the inner malleolus at the level of its most prominent part, anterior to the Achilles tendon	Cough, diaphragm spasm, mouth & throat conditions, toothaches, labor, impotence, inflammation of mammary glands

Important Points on the Kidney Meridian (continued)

Point		Location	Symptoms of Imbalance
K 4 "Water Spring"	Lo Point	½ *cun* slightly posterior and below K 3	Painful heel, impotence, hysteria, crying, premenstrual depression
K 6 "Shining Sea"		1 *cun* directly below internal malleolus	Insomnia, menstrual irregularity, tonsillitis, epilepsy, sore throat, painful or swollen ankle, insect bites
K 10 "Yin Valley"	Water Point	At the medial end of the popliteal (knee) crease, between 2 tendons	Knee pain and weakness, vaginal discharge, disorders of the genitals, genital pain, impotence
K 11 "Transverse Bone"	Penetrating Channel	On the superior border of the pubic bone, ½ *cun* from the midline (CV)	Hernia, impotence, tension in pregnancy, painful penis & scrotum
K 27 "Store-house"		In the depression between the 1st rib and the clavicle, 2 *cun* lateral to the midline (CV)	Chest pain, cough, asthma, vomiting, chaotic meridian flow, low energy in the body

Traditional Indication for Use of Kidney Meridian

Chest problems	Diarrhea	Fear	Sensitivity to cold
Coldness of limbs	Ears ringing	Impotence	Sterility
Cystitis	Edema	Insomnia	Urinary problems
Diabetes	Fatigue	Menstrual disorders	

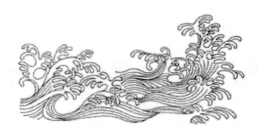

PERICARDIUM MERIDIAN

Base Points:

B 38

P 6

CV 17

Source Point:
P 7

Yin or Yang:
Ying - Zang

Paired Meridian:
Triple Burner

5 Element:
Heart

Time Cycle:
7 P.M. – 9 P.M.

Relationships:
Constructive – Sp/St
Destructive – Lu/Li

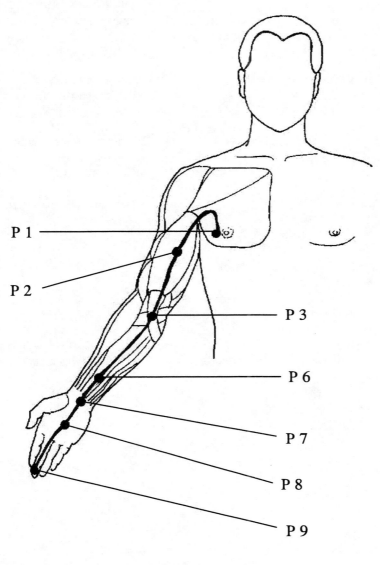

P 1
P 2
P 3
P 6
P 7
P 8
P 9

Important Points on the Pericardium Meridian

Point		Location	Symptoms of Imbalance
P 1 "Heavenly Pond"	Entry Point	1 *cun* lateral to the center of the the nipple, in the 4th intercostal space	Problems with the chest, diaphragm, lymph glands, & breast, mammary pain, insufficient milk
P 2 "Heavenly Spring"		On the inside of the upper arm, at the level of the deltoid V	Coughing, bronchitis, vomiting, anorexia, arm pain, cardiac pain, pulmonary congestion
P 3 "Crooked Marsh"		On the elbow fold in the small hollow, inside (on the ulna side) the tendon of the biceps	Chest pain, arm pain, sterility, irregular periods

Important Points on the Pericardium Meridian (continue)

Point		Location	Symptoms of Imbalance
P 6 "Inner Gate"	Lo Point	2 *cun* above the waist, between the ulna and radius, on the inside of the arm	Nausea, hiccoughs, chest pain, motion sickness, shock, dizziness, epilepsy, insomnia, menstrual irregularity
P 7 "Big Mound"	Source Point	Middle of the wrist crease	Prone to sadness or fear, insomnia, wrist problems, epilepsy, insanity, yin organ disorders
P 8 "Labor Palace"	Exit Point	Middle of the palm, between middle & ring fingers	Wrist pain, writer's cramp, hardening of arteries, indigestion, emotional imbalance
P 9 "Middle Rushing"	Last Point	At the midpoint of the tip of the middle finger, or at the base of the nail on the radial side	Shock, stroke, exhaustion, high fever, epilepsy

Traditional Indication for Use of Pericardium Meridian

Anxiety
Arteriosclerosis
Blurred vision
Bronchitis
Children's nightmares
Cough & fever

Depression
Discord in relationships
Emotional disturbances
Headache
Heart discomfort

Hot palms
Insomnia
Inappropriate laughter
Menstrual problems
Red face

Shock
Skin problems
Speech
Stiff elbow or arm
Swollen underarm

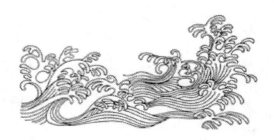

TRIPLE BURNER MERIDIAN

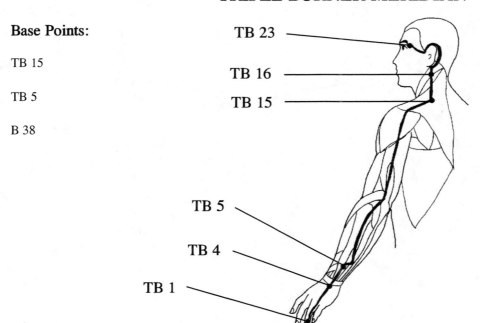

Base Points:

TB 15

TB 5

B 38

TB 23

TB 16

TB 15

TB 5

TB 4

TB 1

Source Point:
TB 4

Yin or Yang:
Yang - Fu

Paired Meridian:
Pericardium

5 Element:
Fire

Time Cycle:
9 P.M. – 11 P.M.

Relationships:
Constructive – Sp/St
Destructive – Lu/Li

Important Points on the Triple Burner Meridian

Point		Location	Symptoms of Imbalance
TB 1 "Gate Rushing"	Entry Point	On the ring finger at the outside corner of the base of the nail	Sore throat, headache, anorexia
TB 4 "Yang Pond"	Source Point	On the dorsal side of the wrist, at the wrist flexure, between the heads of the ulna & radius, & the carpals	Wrist problems, unable to grasp, shivering, diabetes
TB 5 "Outer Gate"	Lo Point	2 *cun* above the wrist crease on the dorsal side, between the ulna & radius	Whole arm painful or swollen, arthritis, stiff neck, toothache, deafness, flu, headache, chest pain, common cold
TB 15 "Heavenly Bone"		On the posterior surface of the shoulder, in a little hollow just above the tip of the scapula	Shoulder & arm pain, stiff neck, fever, low antibody production
TB 16 "Window of Heaven"		Posterior & inferior to the mastoid process	Stiff neck, temporal headache, deafness
TB 23 "Silk Bamboo Hollow"	Exit Point	At the lateral tip of the eyebrow	Eyes twitching or swollen, vision blurred

Traditional Indication for Use of Triple Burner Meridian

Arthritis	Colds	Deafness	Epilepsy	Inflammation	Toothache
Boils	Confusion	Diabetes	Eye problems	Jaw problems	
Bronchitis	Constipation	Diarrhea	Fever	Shoulder pain	
Chills	Cough	Elbow stiffness	Headache	Sweating abnormally	

GALL BLADDER MERIDIAN

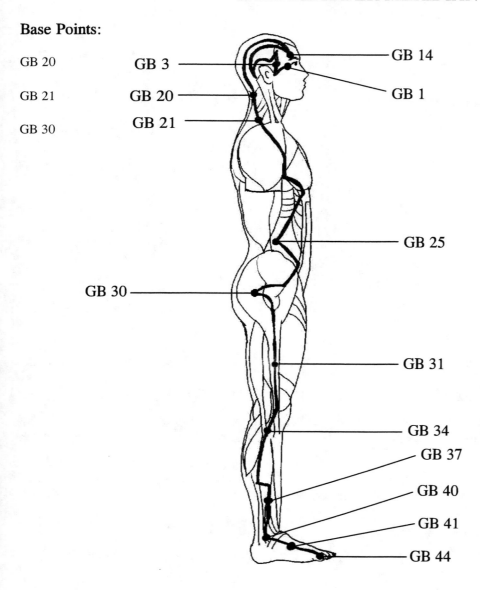

Base Points:

GB 20

GB 21

GB 30

GB 14

GB 3

GB 20

GB 21

GB 1

GB 25

GB 30

GB 31

GB 34

GB 37

GB 40

GB 41

GB 44

Source Point:
GB 40

Yin or Yang:
Yang - Fu

Paired Meridian:
Liver/Yin

5 Element:
Wood

Time Cycle:
11 P.M. – 1 A.M.

Relationships:
Constructive – H/SI
Destructive – Sp/St

Important Points on the Gall Bladder Meridian

Point		Location	Symptoms of Imbalance
GB 1 "Eye Bone"	Entry Point	½ *cun* lateral to the outer corner of the eye in a hollow	Eye problems, conjunctivitis, eyes weak or red, headache, facial paralysis
GB 3 "Upper Gate"	St/GB Reunion Point	Just above the zygomatic arch	Migraines, facial paralysis, ear problems, toothache
GB 14 "Yang White"		On the forehead, 1 *cun* above the middle of the eyebrow	Frontal headache, facial paralysis, glaucoma, poor memory, unclear thinking

Important Points on the Gall Bladder Meridian (continued)

Point		Location	Symptoms of Imbalance
GB 20 "Wind Pond"		Under the occipital ridge, in the hollow between the trapezius & the sternocleidomastoid	Headache, migraine, ear or eye problems, dizziness, stiff neck, shoulder pain, rheumatism
GB 21 "Shoulder Well"		At the base of the neck, just anterior to the trapezius	Back, shoulder, & neck tension, rheumatism, headache, hyperthyroidism, irritability
GB 25 "Capital Bone"	Kidney Alarm Point	Just beyond the tip of the 12th rib	Colic, vomiting, nephritis, lower back pain, fear
GB 30 "Jumping Circle"	GB/B Reunion Point	Posterior to the most prominent part of the trochanter, in the deep hollow. Sensitive point.	Sciatica, frustration, hip problems, rheumatism, paralysis, epilepsy
GB 31 "Wind Market"		On the external surface of the thigh. When standing erect, hands to side, at the tip of the middle finger	Paralysis of lower extremities, sciatica, hip pain
GB 34 "Yang Mound Spring"		On the external surface of the leg below the head of the fibula, between the two muscles	Muscle tightness, lumbago, tight ligaments & tendons, shin splints, knee problems, neurasthenia
GB 37 "Bright Light"	Lo Point	5 *cun* above lateral malleolus, at anterior margin of fibula	Pain in legs, cannot stand for long periods, eye diseases
GB 40 "Wilderness Mound"	Source Point	In the hollow anterior to the external malleolus	Ankle pain, arthritis, sciatica, muscular spasms, sprained ankle
GB 41 "Foot Above Tears"	Exit Point	At the angle of the 4th & 5th metatarsals	Headache, sciatica, ankle pain, irritability, shoulder tension, arthritis, rheumatic pains that move around
GB 44 "Extreme Yin"		Outside corner of the base of the 4th toenail	Headache, dreams of ghosts, insomnia or excessive sleep

Traditional Indication for Use of Bladder Meridian

Ankle pain	Headache	Neck problems	Shoulder problems
Arthritis	Irritable or judgmental	Paralysis	Sighing frequently
Diarrhea	Jaw problems	Sciatica	Stiff muscles
Eye problems	Mental indecision	Sides of body ache	Stiff 4th toe

LIVER MERIDIAN

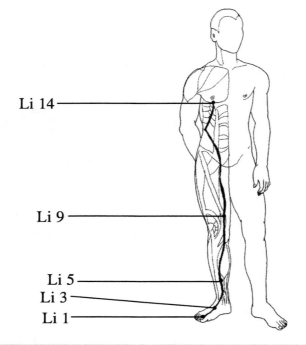

Base Point:

B 42

Source Point:
Li 3

Yin or Yang:
Yin - Zang

Paired Meridian:
Gall Bladder/Yang

5 Element:
Wood

Time Cycle:
1 A.M. – 3 A.M.

Relationships:
Constructive – H/SI
Destructive – Sp/St

Li 14

Li 9

Li 5
Li 3
Li 1

Important Points on the Liver Meridian

Point		Location	Symptoms of Imbalance
Li 1 "Big Heap"	Entry Point	In the lateral corner of the base of the big toenail	Hernia, irregular menstruation, prolapsed uterus
Li 3* "Bigger Rushing"	Source Point	In the angle of the 1st and 2nd metatarsals between the big toe	Master tonic point, foot cramps, tired eyes, headache, allergies, toxicity, hangover, arthritis
*Li 3's are two of the four gates.			
Li 5 "Insect Ditch"	Lo Point	5 *cun* above the medial malleolus in trough between posterior margin of tibia & gastrocnemius muscle	Abdominal pains, retention of urine, pain in scrotum, irregular periods, incontinence of urine, boils on buttocks, toxicity in stomach
Li 9 "Joy of Living"	Detox Point	1/3 of the way up the inside of thigh, between vastus medialis & M. sartorius	Muscular spasms, pain in legs / abdomen irregular periods, incontinence of urine, boils on buttocks, toxicity
Li 14 "Gate of Hope"	Liver Alarm Point, Exit Point	In the intercostal space of the 6th & 7th ribs, directly below the nipple	Hepatitis, chest pain, belching, vomiting sour fluid, difficult delivery, postpartum troubles, hypertension

Traditional Indication for Use of Liver Meridian

Allergies	Digestion problems	Menstrual problems	Planning problems
Depression	(especially of fats)	Muscle spasms, cramps	Repressed anger
Excessive anger	Hernia	Nails cracking, soft	Temper problems
Eye problems	Indecision	Nausea	Urinary problems

Part II:
Practical Application of TCM

使用

方法

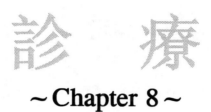

~ Chapter 8 ~

Diagnosis

A healthy body is a balance of the Yin and Yang. The focus is holistic, encompassing delving into the environment, the emotions, and the way of life, or lifestyle, of the client. Illness is generated by one or more factors.

The Environmental Factors

Exterior influences can easily affect the body. The environmental factors, or the "Six Climatic Phenomena," are the Wind, Cold, Fire, Dampness, Dryness, and Summer Heat. They are also called the "Six Evils."

The Emotional Factors

According to the *Nei Jing*, the seven emotional factors of joy, anger, sadness, grief, pensiveness, fear, and fright can influence the body's harmony. If they become imbalanced either as an excess or deficiency over a long period of time, a person's health suffers. The *Nei Jing* states that "excess joy is associated with slow and scattered Chi; excess anger induces the Chi to ascend; excess sadness and grief weakens the Chi; excess pensiveness generates 'knottedness' or 'stuckness'; fear results in descending Chi; and fright induces chaotic Chi."

The Way of Life Factors

These are neither external nor internal factors and are called one's lifestyle in the West. The factors include diet, sexual activity, and physical activity.

Other Factors included are burns, bites, parasites, and trauma.

The Four Examinations

Diagnosis has Four Stages of Examinations to recognize the signs and symptoms of imbalance. These are: Looking (observing that which is visible); Listening (to the voice and respiration) and Smelling; Asking (specific questions); and Touching (taking the pulse).

Looking

The practitioner will observe the:
1. General appearance, which includes the physical shape, manners, behavior, and state of *Shen*
2. Facial color
3. Quality of the eyes
4. Bodily secretions and excretions; and
5. Tongue, which includes the materials of the tongue itself, the coating of the tongue, its shape and movement. This is the second most important examination.

Fig 8A. Correspondence of tongue areas to Organs   Fig. 8B. Correspondence of face areas to Organs

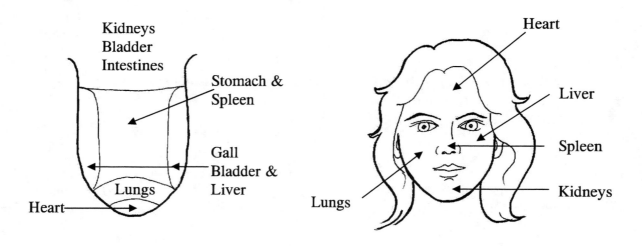

Fig. 8C. Correspondence of eye areas to Organs

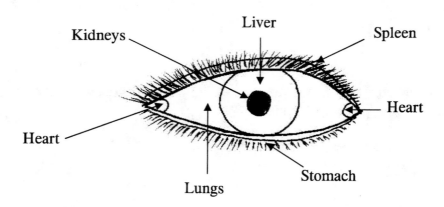

Listening and Smelling

This examination includes the:
1. Voice and respiration of the client; and
2. Bodily odors (either a foul, rotten, and nauseating smell, which usually indicates Heat and/or Excess, or a pungent fishy smell that may hurt the nose, which indicates Cold and/or Deficiency)

Asking

This is more extensive than simply taking a medical history. Important questions include: sensations of cold or hot; perspiration; headaches and dizziness; urination and stool; thirst; appetite and tastes; sleep; gynecological concerns; and quality and location of pain.

Touching

The examination of touching by taking a pulse is the most important examination. The art of pulse taking requires thorough training, great experience, and the gift of sensitivity. There are around twenty-four to thirty pulse types. The quality of the type of the pulse is determined by its depth, speed, width, strength, overall shape, quality, rhythm, and length.

Fig. 8D. Chinese Pulse Taking Method adapted from *The Web That Has No Weaver: Understanding Chinese Medicine*, by Ted J. Kaptchuk

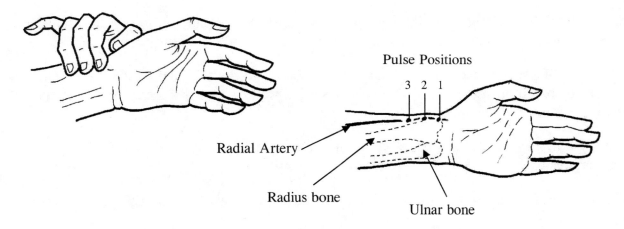

Corresponding Relationships of Pulse Positions and Organs

Position	Left Wrist	Right Wrist
First	Heart	Lungs
Second	Liver	Spleen
Third	Kidney Yin	Kidney Yang (Life-gate line)

Measurement

The Chinese measurement of the body is called *cun*. One *cun* is the width of the person's thumb. And three *cun* is the width of the first, middle, fourth, and little fingers put together.

Fig. 8E. Finger Measurements

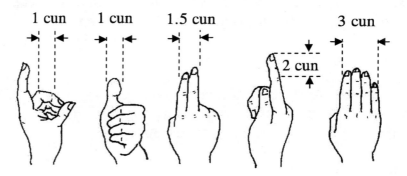

Identification of Patterns

Identification of patterns is the process of identifying the basic disharmony that underlies all clinical manifestations. Rather than analyzing the symptoms and signs one by one in trying to find a cause for them as Western medicine does, Chinese medicine forms an overall picture, taking all the symptoms and signs into consideration to identify the underlying disharmony.

There are several methods used to identify the patterns. These are used in different situations and were formulated over time in the development of TCM. The various identifying patterns are:

1. Identification of the patterns by Eight Principles based on the four pairs of polar oppositions: Yin and Yang, Exterior and Interior, Excess and Deficiency, and Cold and Hot.

2. Identification of the basic disharmony of Chi, Blood, and Body Fluids: such as deficiency, stagnation, or rebelliousness of Chi; deficiency, stasis, heat, or loss of Blood; and deficiency of Fluids, edema, and phlegm.

3. Identification by the Internal Organs based on the pathological changes occurring in the Internal Organs.

4. Identification by the Pathogenic Factors. These patterns deal mostly with the Exterior influences.

5. Identification by the Five Elements according to the generating, overacting, and controlling sequences of the Five Elements.

6. Identification by the Channels or Meridians according to the symptoms and signs related to each channel rather than the Organ.

7. Identification by the Six Stages to treat the exterior Cold and interior Hot.

8. Identification by the Four Levels of the exterior Wind-Heat.

9. Identification by the Three Burners. This method is used with the previous one for diagnosis and treatment of feverish infectious diseases starting with the invasion of Wind-Heat.

Main Excess/Deficiency and Heat/Cold Signs

General Signs	Tongue	Pulse
Excess Patterns Ponderous, heavy movement; heavy, coarse respiration; pressure and touch increase discomfort	thick moss	strong (full, wiry, slippery, etc.)
Deficiency Patterns Frail, weak movement; tiredness; shortness of breath; pressure relieves discomfort; inactive; passive appearance; low voice; dizziness; little appetite	pale material; thin moss	weak (empty, frail, almost non-existent, etc.)
Heat Patterns Red face; high fever; dislike of heat; cold reduces discomfort; rapid movement; outgoing manner; thirst or desire for cold drinks; dark urine; constipation	red material; yellow moss	rapid
Cold Patterns Pale, white face; limbs cold; fear of cold; heat reduces discomfort; slow movement; withdrawn manner; no thirst or a desire for hot drinks	pale material; white moss	slow

Yin and Yang

Yin   =   Interior + Deficient + Cold
Yang =   Exterior + Excess   + Hot

Signs of Yin and Yang Patterns

Examination	Yin Signs	Yang Signs
Looking	quiet; withdrawn; slow, frail manner; client is tired and weak, likes to lie down curled up; no spirit; excretions and secretions are watery and thin; tongue material is pale, puffy, and moist; tongue moss is thin and white	agitated, restless, active manner; rapid, forceful movement; red face; client likes to stretch when lying down; tongue material is red or scarlet, and dry; tongue moss is yellow and thick
Listening and Smelling	voice is low and without strength; few words; respiration is shallow and weak; shortness of breath; acrid odor	voice is coarse, rough, and strong; client is talkative; respiration is full and deep; putrid odor
Asking	feels cold; reduced appetite; no taste in mouth; desires warmth and touch; copious and clear urine; pressure relieves discomfort; scanty, pale menses	client feels hot; dislikes heat; constipation; scanty, dark urine; dry mouth; thirst
Touching	frail, almost non-existent, thin, empty, or otherwise weak pulse	full, rapid, slippery, wiry, floating, or otherwise strong pulse

Qualities of Pain

Quality of Pain	Signification
Diminished by heat	Cold
Diminished by cold	Heat
Relieved by touch or pressure	Deficiency
Aggravated by touch or pressure	Excess
Diminished after eating	Deficiency
Increased after eating	Excess
Increases in humid weather	Dampness
Accompanied by bloating or sense of fullness	Stagnant Chi
Sharp and stabbing, fixed in one location	Congealed Blood
Sensation of heaviness	Dampness
Moves from place to place	Wind of Stagnant Chi
Slight and accompanied by fatigue	Deficient Chi or Dampness

In addition to your good interviewing and diagnostics skills, palpating of the Yu points mentioned in Chapter 7 and your intuition will be combined during an evaluation to come to some conclusion about how you will proceed with your client. Equally as important is what you personally bring to a session—your biases, fears, stresses, intentions, attitude, state of mind (either upset or joyful). Awareness and compassion are the key ingredients to offering help to your clients. Refer to Chapter 10 (Self-Help Exercises) for aids in achieving balanced Chi in yourself.

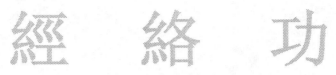

~ Chapter 9 ~

Meridian Body Therapy

Meridian Body Therapy is based on acupuncture, Tui Na, and Shiatsu concepts. Unlike acupuncture, which uses needles, Meridian Body Therapy applies stimulation, in the form of pressure, on specific points and specific energy pathways along the acupuncture meridians. Pressure is usually applied with the fingers, knuckles, thumbs, hands (open or closed), arms, elbows, and sometimes the feet. Stress within the body can be caused by many factors, including illness, injury, and emotional upset, all of which can result in congestion in acupuncture points. Muscular tension also tends to accumulate around acupuncture points, causing blockages in the flow of vital energy. Applying pressure to various points correlating to different meridians and acupuncture points can help the body restore the flow of Chi and balance itself. Prolonged pressure on acupressure points may release endorphins that help to control pain, as has been proven to happen with stimulation by acupuncture. Meridian Body Therapy, like acupressure point bodywork, can be used for preventive health care for clients. It can also be used for self-help, and this will be explored in the next chapter. For now we will concentrate on helping clients relax and on stimulating the flow of Chi in specific meridian points.

Traditionally, Meridian Body Therapy is done on the floor on a mat; however, all the techniques shown can also be done while the client is lying on a massage table or in a sitting position. Most of the techniques can be used in all the Meridian Body Therapy routines. You can be creative with the routines by using various techniques discussed below as you see fit.

Refer to chapter 7 for the positions of the meridians and the locations of the acupuncture points. Use the soothing techniques of palming along the meridians at the beginning of the routines to induce a state of relaxation in your client before using any of the more focusing techniques like thumbing or *An Fa* for more specific work.

Some of the common techniques used in Meridian Body Therapy

Palming
Use either one or both palms—flat palms pressing or alternating pressure. Come from the center, and use your body weight instead of your arm strength.

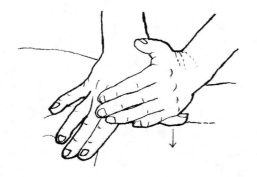

Thumbing

Can use one or both thumbs. Apply the pad of the thumb for soothing touch and the tip for more penetrating pressure. There are several methods of thumbing such as static pressure, alternating pressure, reinforced thumb (as shown in drawing), circular thumbing, and so forth.

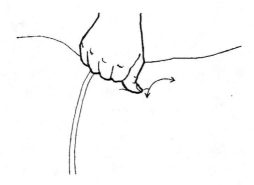

An Fa (One-finger Manipulation)

Press on one point, and rock the thumb back and forth rhythmically. Wrist, arm, and shoulders should be relaxed; no jerking. Can be done with either one or both thumbs.

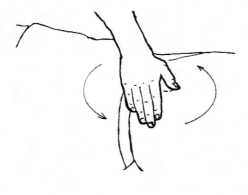

Mo Fa (Palm or Palms Rubbing)

Using one or two palms, rub gently in circular motion. Keep wrist, arm, and shoulders relaxed.

Scraping

In slow motion press deeply into affected area, and scrape downward or side-to-side. Do in very small range of distance—approximately ¼ inch.

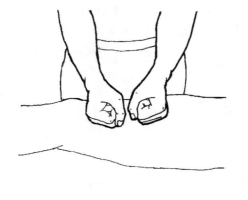

Beating with Fists

Can be either with open, loose fists or with closed, firm fists (as shown). Keep arms and shoulders relaxed. Let the wrists do most of the work. Use loose fists on tender areas such as inner thighs.

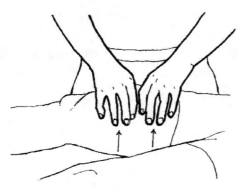

Plucking

Using both hands, grab as many muscles as you can and lift, shake, and release slowly or quickly.

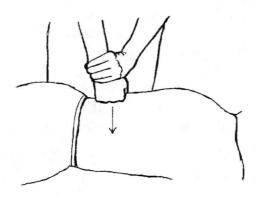

An Fa with Fist

Can use either one, supported (as shown), both, or alternating fists. Use the flat area of the fist, and compress for about 1 to 2 seconds and release. Do not press on one area repeatedly; move up and down the muscles. Use proper body mechanics and come from your body weight and your center.

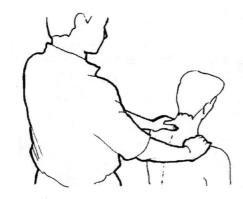

Grasping

Use hands to grasp or pinch firmly but gently. Client will feel relaxed yet stimulated at the same time. This technique is done mostly on major muscles groups, such as the trapezius muscles.

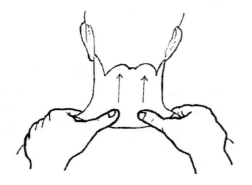

Thumb Kneading

Move thumbs back and forth in a circular kneading fashion up and down the muscles. Usually done along the neck muscles.

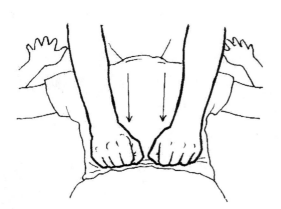

Fist/Hand/Palm Stroking

Can do in one direction or can alternate strokes, using hands, fists (as shown), or palms. Should be firm and smooth yet relaxed and warming. Repeat as many times as you see fit.

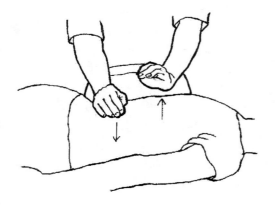

Pai Fa

Along the surface area where you are working, cup your hands and beat in an up-and-down motion. The technique should be rapid but not heavy or pounding. It can produce stimulation ranging from light to strong. The emphasis is on the upward motion.

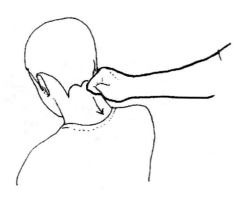

Knuckle Stroking

Usually done on the neck. Start from the base of the skull on the neck, and stroke down, using the knuckles of the fist as shown. Repeat several times.

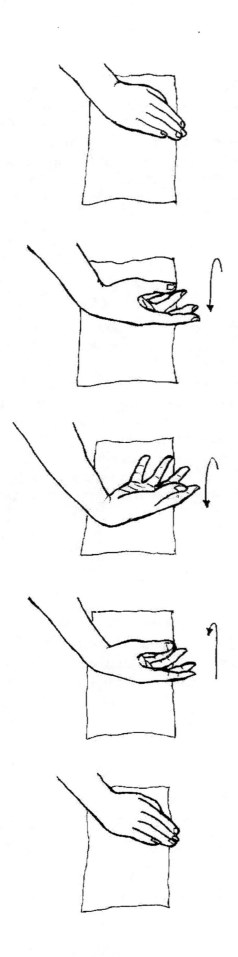

Rolling

This is one of the main techniques of Tui Na and can take a while to learn. So be patient, and go slow at the beginning and relax. There should not be any discomfort. If you feel any discomfort, you are not doing it correctly.

Relax your hand, wrist, arm, shoulders, and body to perform this technique.

Start by placing your hand with palm flat and relaxed on the muscles. Using the 5th metacarpalphalangeal joint as the pivoting point, roll your hand to the back side, reaching a hyperflexion with your whole back of the hand on the muscles without compromising your wrist.

Return your hand to the starting position, applying the same pressure throughout the whole movement. Go slowly in the beginning while learning this technique, and go faster as you get comfortable with the movement and hand manipulation.

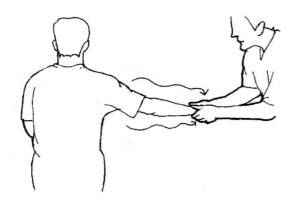

Shaking
Rapidly, yet gently and rhythmically, shake one arm in a wave-like motion while pulling in traction. The shake should travel from the wrist up to the shoulder, affecting the wrist, elbow, arm, and shoulder.

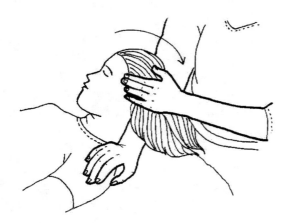

Neck Rotation and Stretching
Place your right hand on the left shoulder with your arm across and under the neck. Raise the head with your right arm while doing the rotation and stretching as shown. Then, let the head roll to the opposite side by lowering your right arm, guiding with your left hand. Return the head to the starting position, and repeat the whole process on the opposite side.

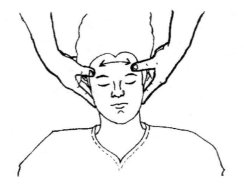

Tui Fa
Using the pads of your thumbs, stroke firmly and smoothly across the area being worked on. This is done across smaller areas like the forehead, face, neck, etc.

6-Step Basic Routine for Calming Your Client (client in prone position)

1. **Leaning Palms** — With your fingers extended, place your hands on both sides of the spine. Breathe in, and on exhaling, apply pressure through your hands. Move down the back until you reach the sacrum. This is done firmly yet gently. Avoid placing hands directly on the spine.

2. **Cat's Paw** — Positioning is the same as Leaning Palms, except alternate the pressure between your hands. This technique can be applied over the whole back and down the legs in any pattern.

3. **Diagonal Stretch** — Position yourself on the side of your client, crossing your forearms, and place your upper hand on the base of the shoulder blade located on the opposite side of where you are. At the same time, place your lower hand at the top of the iliac crest on your side. Lean forward, stretching the client's back diagonally. Switch hands, and stretch the opposite side.

4. **Rocking Fists** — Make soft fists with both hands. Place your fists at the space between the 12th rib and the iliac crest. Roll your fists.

5. **Tiger's Mouth** — Placing one hand on the client's sacrum or shoulder, slowly move your other hand down the leg or arm. Apply 80% compression and 20% rotation to make a press and twisting motion.

6. **God Makes a Snake** — Place one hand above the knee, and the other below, and "roll" the leg medially and laterally, while spreading your hands to the distal and proximal ends of the leg.

Pressure Guidelines

When applying pressure to an acupressure point, light to deep pressure is applied on the point no more than one minute, or until you feel a pulsating sensation under your finger. You can use your palm, thumb, index, or middle finger, or any of the appropriate techniques shown above to apply pressure throughout the routines.

Step-by-Step Routines for Applying Techniques to Specific Meridians

Working the Lung and Large Intestine Meridians

1. Perform the 6-Step Basic Routine for Calming Your Client.
2. Relax in a kneeling position, with your client in the supine position; rest your palm on his/her Hara, the energy center believed to be 2" below the navel and inside the abdomen in front of the spine. Pay attention to his/her breathing. Generally, breathing gets deeper as the client relaxes.
3. Rotate and stretch the right arm, exploring its full range of motion; then place it at a 45° angle to the client's side with the palm facing up.

4. Placing your right palm on his/her shoulder and your left hand on the arm, use the Tiger's Mouth technique down the arm to the wrist.
5. From the wrist continue down the thumb by squeezing the pad of the client's thumb, with your thumb and index finger, as you work to the end of the thumb.
6. Repeat as often as you like in order to stimulate the meridian.
7. Work specific point locations down the arm, using L 1, 5, 7, 9, 10, & 11.
8. Rotate the arm medially to begin working the LI meridian, and perform the Tiger's Mouth technique down the arm to the wrist.
9. When you reach the forearm, use your thumb to massage points along the line of the index finger.
10. Repeat as often as you like in order to stimulate the meridian.
11. Work specific point locations down the arm, using LI 1, 4, 5, 6, 11, 14, & 20.
12. For further relaxation, end by applying traction and jostling and by brushing the arm.
13. Repeat the process on the left arm.

Working the Stomach and Spleen Meridians

1. With your client supine, move to a kneeling position with his/her head in between your knees. You do not want to kneel so close that your client feels oppressed.
2. With a relaxed state of mind, lean with both hands onto your client's shoulders.
3. Loosen your client's neck by holding your hands on either side over the ears and temples for a few minutes, and then roll the head gently from side to side or use the Neck Rotation and Stretching technique shown in the technique section of this chapter.
4. Move your hands to the base of the skull. Lean back, and your client's head should lift gently from the floor. Roll the client's head onto one hand and then the other. This provides you access to work the Stomach meridian points on the opposite side of the face.
5. Once you have worked these points, apply gentle pressure with the palm of your hand down the neck to the shoulders and laterally to the deltoids.
6. Repeat on the other side of the neck.
7. Once you have completed the work on the head for the Stomach meridian, position yourself to work on either leg.
8. Perform the Tiger's Mouth technique down the lateral side of the leg.
9. Work the Stomach meridian by rolling the leg medially, and place your lower foot on the client's leg or foot in order to stabilize it. Then palm down the meridian again.
10. Stay in this position, and thumb your way down the meridian about one finger-width inside the shinbone.
11. When you reach the foot of the client, remove your stabilizing foot from the client and thumb along the line of the second toe.
12. At the end of the second toe, apply a gentle traction.
13. Now work the specific points along the leg.
14. Stretch the client's leg by bringing the knee to the chest, and then slowly rotate the leg in a circle, exploring the range of motion.
15. Now rotate your client's leg laterally with the knee slightly bent, and let it rest either on your knee or a pillow.
16. Use the Cat's Paw technique to palm the medial aspect from the thigh down to the ankle.

17. Thumb down the Spleen meridian approximately two finger-widths medial to the patella. This can be a tender area, so move slowly.
18. Work the points along the Spleen meridian from the toes, going up the body toward the head.
19. Repeat #7 through #18 on the other leg.

Working the Heart and Small Intestine Meridians

1. Perform the 6-Step Basic Routine for Calming Your Client.
2. Put your client in a prone position with his/her hand (one closest to you) in a 90° angle to the body. Place your inside hand above the heart area on your client's back.
3. Turn your client's hand so that the palm is facing up, exposing the inner part of the arm.
4. From the armpit, thumb or palm down the arm to the wrist; then thumb down the lateral aspect of the 5th finger.
5. Repeat step #4, using the thumb at a more penetrating angle.
6. Apply pressure to specific points on the Heart meridian.
7. Place your support hand on your client's back on the opposite side from where you are working.
8. Thumb the Small Intestine meridian from the back of the neck down to the shoulder blade. Do this 3 times on each side.
9. Using the edge of your hand, lean forward to apply steady pressure on the Small Intestine meridian over the scapula and out to the arm. You may also use your fingers and thumbs.
10. Remain in contact with your client as you move to his/her side. Move the arm out a little and on its edge so that the little finger is facing up.
11. Palm the arm downward from the armpit. Leave your other hand on the shoulder blade. As you reach below the elbow, either continue the palming or thumb down to the wrist if that is easier for you.
12. Repeat #11 with a more penetrating pressure.
13. Continue to work the meridian on the 5th finger by squeezing with your index finger and thumb.
14. Apply pressure to specific points on the Small Intestine meridian.
15. When finished, gently pick up the arm at the wrist and shoulder. Lift and apply traction to the shoulder. Move the arm away from the ribs, and rotate the shoulder.
16. Place one palm between the shoulder blade and spine, with the other hand under the same shoulder. Pick up the shoulder, forcing the shoulder blade over your other hand. This is scapular distraction, which is very potent for relaxing the shoulder.
17. Finish working on the arm by brushing it.
18. Repeat steps #10 - #17 on the other arm.

Working the Bladder and Kidney Meridians

1. With your client prone, perform the Leaning Palms and Cat's Paw techniques down the back in the area between the shoulder blades.
2. The Bladder meridian has two main branches down the back between the shoulder blades. The first is 1½ finger-widths from the spine and the second is 3 finger-widths from the spine. Thumb down this general area from the top of the shoulders to the pelvis.
3. Go to either side of your client and work the opposite side of his/her back, providing lateral pressure. Allow your hands to sink into the muscles, and then slowly lean into your client's back. Work from either the top or bottom of the back.

4. From this position provide the same pressure, using your elbows on the side of the client's back that is closest to you. Move slowly when applying pressure, and be careful of the pressure you exert over the kidney area.

5. From the lateral side of the hip to the top of the thigh, work the gluteal muscles with your fists.

6. Apply pressure into the edge of the sacrum. Follow the border of the sacrum to the pelvis and then to the lateral portion of the hip. This can be done bilaterally or only to one side at a time.

7. Returning to the shoulders, begin thumbing down the back from the top of the shoulders to the iliac crest at the top of the pelvis. Be careful as you work the kidney areas. Avoid quick, piercing pressure over the kidneys. Then work back up in the opposite direction.

8. Moving to the legs, work downward, using the Tiger's Mouth technique. Place the heel of the hand directly over the meridian that runs down the center of the leg.

9. Thumb down this part of the leg. Follow the meridian to the bottom of the gastrocnemius where it deviates laterally and then again runs straight down to behind the lateral malleolus and down the lateral side of the foot.

10. Work the specific Bladder points, and then repeat the above process on the other leg.

11. Turn your client over. Position yourself to perform the Tiger's Mouth technique down either leg. Rotate the leg laterally to gain access to the inner thigh and leg.

12. Face and work the opposite leg. Thumb down the Kidney meridian that runs along the medial thigh; then move down the medial side of the lower leg, continuing down the medial ankle, ending at the center of the foot. Locate and thumb the specific points on the Kidney meridian.

13. Move to the other side, and perform steps #11 & #12 on the other leg.

14. Perform leg stretches.

15. Stimulate the Kidney meridian points on the anterior side of the upper body.

Working the Pericardium and Triple Burner Meridians

1. With your client on his/her side, place a pillow under the head, and, for support, place the client's top leg in front of his/her other leg.

2. Position yourself at the client's back. Insert your arm under the client's armpit. Clasp the shoulder with both hands, and begin to move it slowly in circles. Use your body movement to follow and feel the limits of the motion, and rotate the joint more widely. Rotate the shoulder in both directions.

3. Place your palms on the side of the head that is facing upward. Lean forward, and gently apply pressure through your palms.

4. Thumb from the end of the eyebrow to the front of the ear, then around the ear, and down the back of the neck. To keep your client's head and neck open for work, gently push the shoulder down with your free hand.

5. As you work down to release the tension in the back of the neck, press firmly into the base of the skull and work toward the shoulder.

6. Move to your client's head, and face his/her feet. Placing one palm on the side of the head, thumb with the other hand from the base of the neck to the end of the shoulder.

7. Move to your client's back again. Take his/her arm, and position it so you can access the palm side of the arm.

8. Thumb down the Pericardium meridian, beginning with the bicep.

9. Apply pressure to each point along the meridian.

10. Rotate and place your client's arm so that the palm is facing down. Thumb down the general area of the Triple Burner that runs 2 finger-widths from the medial aspect of the arm and down the middle.
11. Continue toward the space between the knuckles on the 4th and 5th fingers, and finish by squeezing the sides of the 4th finger.
12. Now work the points on the Triple Burner meridian.
13. Repeat steps #1 - #12 on the other side.
14. Turn your client onto his/her back, and apply alternating pressure to the top of his/her shoulders.
15. Move your client's head toward his/her right shoulder. Stop when the shoulder naturally starts to lower.
16. Crossing your arms, stretch the neck laterally by placing your right arm on the top of the left shoulder and your left palm on the right side of the head. Apply pressure with your right hand placed on the shoulder while the left hand simply holds the head gently in position.
17. Reversing your hands, stretch the right shoulder by repeating steps #15 & #16.
18. Lastly, cradle the head with your right palm below the base of the skull and with your left hand placed on the forehead. Hold this pose for several minutes, and have your client take deep breaths.

Working the Gall Bladder and Liver Meridians

1. With your client on his/her side, place a pillow under the head, and, for support, place the client's top leg in front of his/her other leg.
2. Place your palms on the side of the head that is facing upward. Lean forward, and gently apply pressure through your palms.
3. Thumb down the neck with firm pressure from the base of the skull to the shoulder area to release tension in the back of the neck.
4. Work the Gall Bladder meridian points on the head and neck only.
5. Now work the Gall Bladder points on the leg and feet only.
6. Move to your client's hip, and get into a lunge position with your lower leg over the client's straight leg. Place your upper hand on his/her hip, and palm down the lateral aspect of the leg with the other hand.
7. Thumb down the Gall Bladder meridian. Note: If your client has sciatic pain, this may be too painful. Follow the meridian down the lateral side of the thigh and leg, then down the anterior side of the ankle and down the area of the 4th toe. Gently pull the 4th toe.
8. Next, thumb down the Liver meridian along the middle of the inner thigh to the knee. Work to the crease in the knee, and follow down the medial aspect of the leg and down the top of the foot to the great toe.
9. Work the specific Liver points.
10. Repeat the entire process on the client's other side.

99

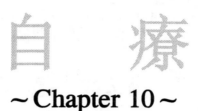

~ Chapter 10 ~

Self-Help Exercises

Chi / Qi Gong

*C*hi Gong is the study and cultivation of Chi and the art of integrating the body with nature. Chi can be anything from the air we breathe in to vital energy. Gong means to work or to train physically over a long period of time. Therefore, Chi Gong can be best understood simply as breath training. There are many styles of Chi Gong, yet all forms of exercises or training that work with one's energy/life force/breath/Chi can be broadly included under Chi Gong. It is a method generally used to strengthen one's internal organs in order to strengthen one's body and mind and a method to cultivate the body, vital energy, and spirit through the disciplines of movement, breath control, and meditation. The ultimate goal of this is enlightenment and immortality.

The Three Major Categories of Chi Gong

There have been countless styles and techniques of Chi Gong practiced throughout China's long history, but the three major categories are:

1. Medical Chi Gong: A branch of TCM used as a therapy for curing illnesses, treating chronic diseases, and healing with Chi by restoring a harmonious balance within the physical body, mind, spirit, and nature. Performed on a regular basis, Chi Gong can be used to stay healthy and prevent illness.
2. Martial Chi Gong: Physical exercise used to develop internal force, to strengthen muscles, build endurance, and for self-defense.
3. Spiritual Chi Gong: Is used for the goal of enlightenment. Chi and breathing exercises along with meditation are the means of reaching harmony and order within one's self and in the universe.

All three types of Chi Gong overlap, and the three form a complete system of energy work. Chi Gong training enables one to build up a reserve of Chi in the body, bringing with it health, vitality, and energy that can be used for healing, spiritual development, and self-defense. Martial arts training benefits health through increasing power while serving as a discipline for spiritual development. Likewise, spiritual cultivation has many health benefits. No matter the form studied, the purpose is to cultivate Chi for health, longevity, and spiritual enlightenment.

Two General Categories

Chi Gong exercise therapy includes both active and passive training. All practices are divided into either *Wai Dan Gong* (external elixir) and *Nei Dan Gong* (internal elixir).

1. *Nei Dan Gong* – Passive Training = motionless = standing, sitting, reclining forms of meditation.
2. *Wai Dan Gong* – Active Training = active = steps = forms of *Kung Fu*, *Tai Ji Chuan,* or other styles of martial arts.

In *Nei Dan Gong* practices there is no outward movement of the body. These practices include postures of meditation. In *Nei Dan Gong,* while the body is still, practitioners rely on intention and breathing, rather than movement, to generate Chi. *Nei Dan Gong* recognizes three energy centers in the body that correspond to the root, solar plexus/heart, and third-eye chakras of Ayurvedic medicine. *Nei Dan* practices are generally considered more advanced.

Wai Dan Gong involves dynamic or moving exercises to build up energy in the limbs and smooth the circulation of Chi through the meridians. *Wai Dan Gong* includes active meditation. *Tai Ji Chuan* serves both as a method of Chi Gong meditation and of self-defense. There are literally hundreds of forms of *Wai Dan Gong*.

The Three Regulations of Chi Gong

Regardless of the style of Chi Gong one practices, the principle of "the three regulations" must be observed. That is, regulation of the body, regulation of the breath, and regulation of the mind.

Regulating the body means finding the middle way between extremes in diet, rest, and exercise in order to build good physical health. It also refers to understanding the correct principles of movement in one's chosen Chi Gong exercise. Proper posture in alignment with gravity and good body mechanics are essential to the flow of Chi.

Regulation of the breath is the bridge between the mind and body. Breath is the most vital link we have with Chi. Control of the breath brings the mind and emotions under control as one's mental state is reflected in one's breathing. Different types of breathing affect the circulation of Chi in different ways. Collecting Chi through proper breath control is essential in all forms of Chi Gong and the martial arts.

Regulation of the mind is the key to success with any Chi Gong practice. When the mind is quiet and fixed, an inner clarity of being emerges. Success in Chi Gong practice is in direct proportion to one's ability to focus the mind, and meditation is the final stage of Chi cultivation. In this clarity body, mind, spirit, and universe become one.

Chi Gong Exercises

Below is just one routine of the many Chi Gong exercises.

Chi Gong For Health

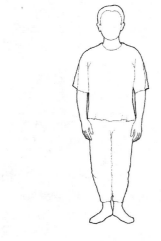

Stand relaxed with heels touching and toes pointing away from the midline, forming a "V."
Shoulders relaxed
Tongue lightly touching the upper palette
Chin tucked in slightly
Breathe naturally.

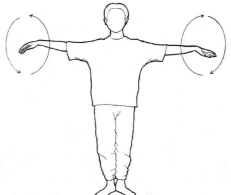

Raise arms.
Rotate backwards - two rotations.

Hands in front of body
Push hands with wrist over wrist in front of body.
Lower body as hands flip and palms are facing up.
Slowly stand up and open arms to both sides.
Rotate backwards - two rotations.

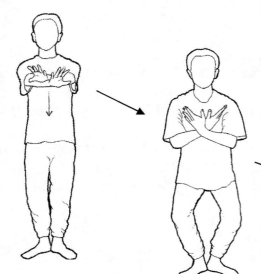

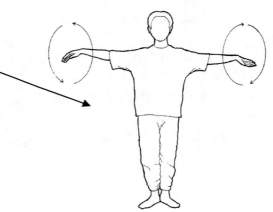

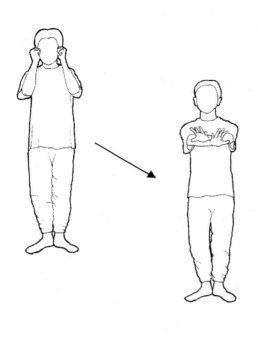

Form a fist with each hand.
Move thumbs toward temples on both sides.
Touch temples with sides of thumbs.
Push hands out in front of body with wrists touching.
Slightly lower the body (still with heels touching).
Open arms upwards while standing up slowly.
Rotate backwards - two rotations.

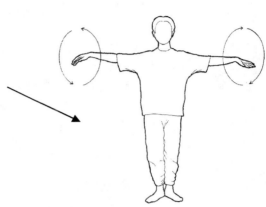

Form a fist with each hand & position thumbs straight out. Move thumbs toward temples.
Extend fingers (fingertips touch).
Flip hands over (palms up).
Stretch up (fingertips touch).
Hands stretch out and down on both sides in a big circle.
Fingers touch in front of the waist area (palms up).

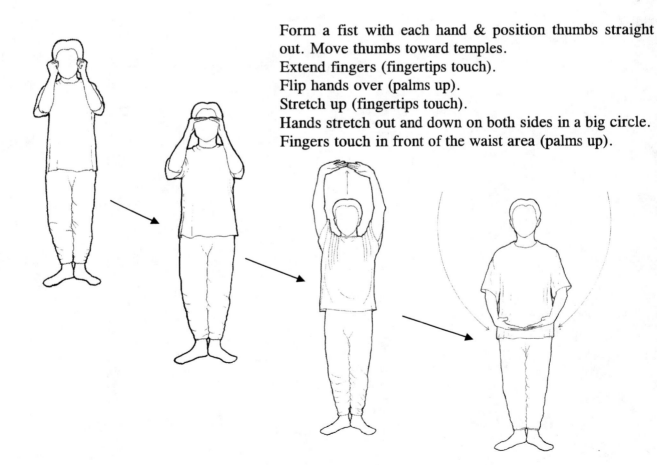

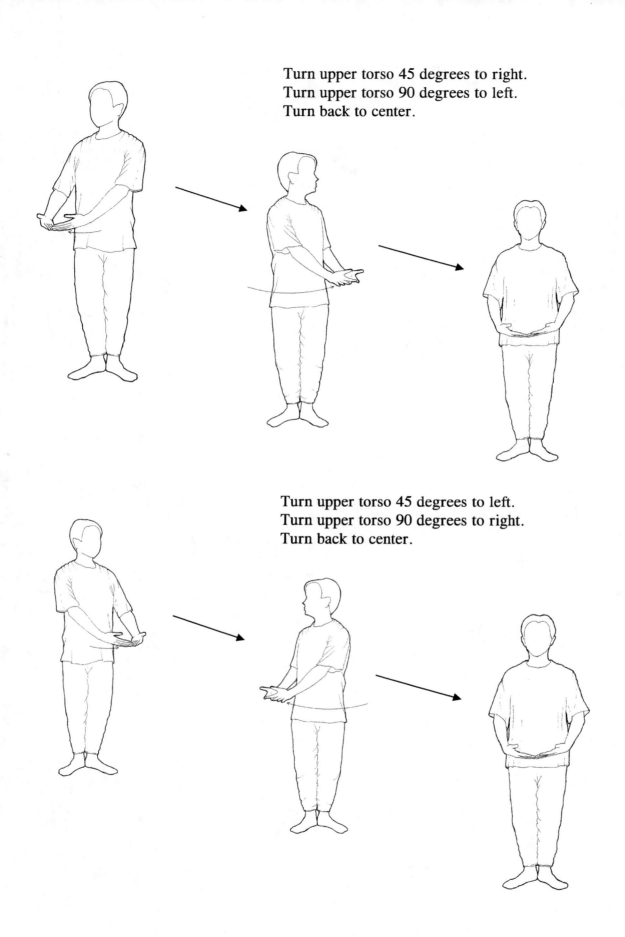

Turn upper torso 45 degrees to right.
Turn upper torso 90 degrees to left.
Turn back to center.

Turn upper torso 45 degrees to left.
Turn upper torso 90 degrees to right.
Turn back to center.

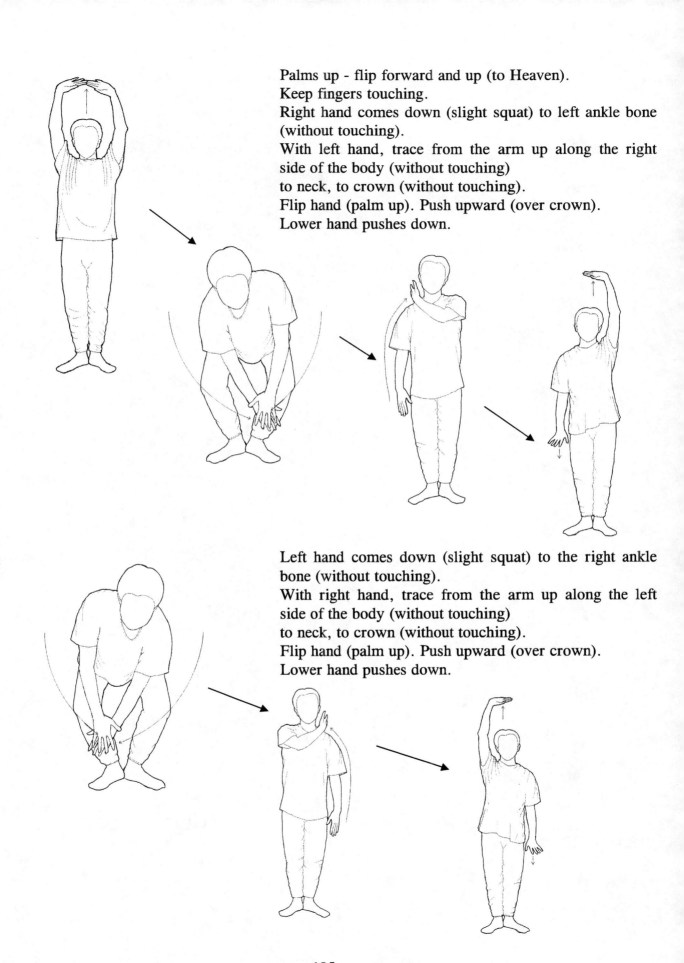

Palms up - flip forward and up (to Heaven).
Keep fingers touching.
Right hand comes down (slight squat) to left ankle bone (without touching).
With left hand, trace from the arm up along the right side of the body (without touching)
to neck, to crown (without touching).
Flip hand (palm up). Push upward (over crown).
Lower hand pushes down.

Left hand comes down (slight squat) to the right ankle bone (without touching).
With right hand, trace from the arm up along the left side of the body (without touching)
to neck, to crown (without touching).
Flip hand (palm up). Push upward (over crown).
Lower hand pushes down.

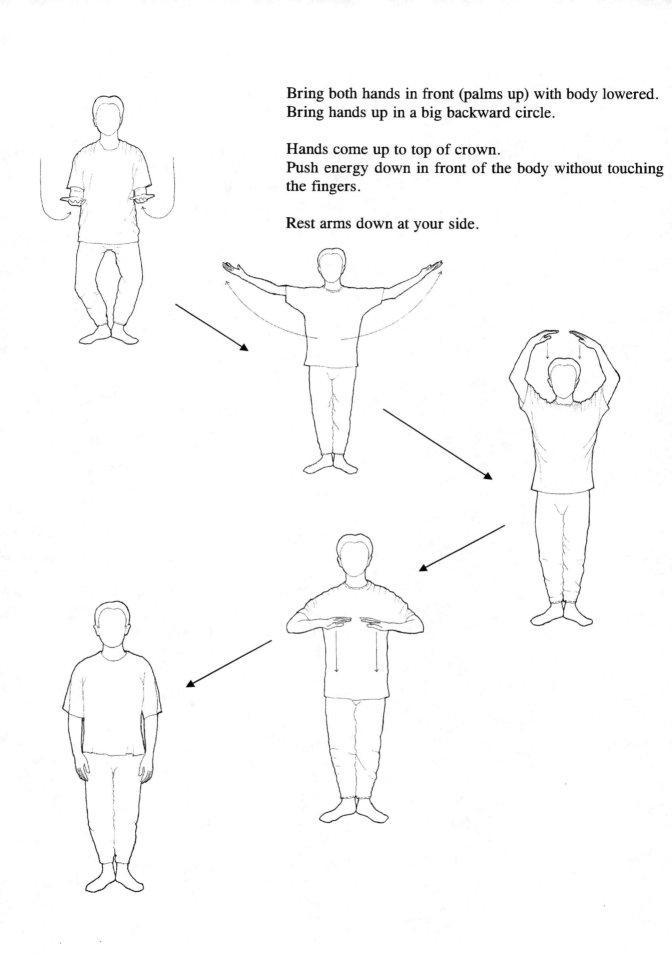

Bring both hands in front (palms up) with body lowered.
Bring hands up in a big backward circle.

Hands come up to top of crown.
Push energy down in front of the body without touching the fingers.

Rest arms down at your side.

Meridian Body Therapy For Self-Help

Meridian Body Therapy can be used in your own preventive health care program and for self-help when problems arise. The four-part routine involves stretching of the meridians and general relaxation work on the musculature. You will probably discover you have been doing some of these techniques naturally already.

Part One – Loosening Your Face, Head, Neck, and Shoulders

1. Sitting or standing, rub your hands together until they are hot. Place your hands over your eyes. Open your eyes, and begin rubbing your face and the top of your head. Work from your chin to the back of your head, and repeat nine times or until your face is warm and relaxed.
2. Place the fingers of both hands just below your eyes and begin stroking under the eyes, massaging the tissue and the bones beneath your skin. Start under the eyes and work to the jaw and up to your hairline.
3. Grasp your nose with the fingers of both hands, loosening up the area between your eyebrows to the tip of your nose.
4. Again, cover your eyes with your fingers, and apply gentle pressure.
5. Begin to palm your forehead on both sides, working from the side of your head to the top. To work the back of your head, lace your fingers behind your head and squeeze the back of your head. Continue past the base of the skull down the neck.
6. Using your fingers, rub the area at the base of the skull.
7. Place your thumbs at the base of the skull. Move your thumbs in a circular motion. You can work into the base of the skull and directly into the side of the neck.
8. From here, work the region of your hairline to the front of your head with your thumbs.
9. Place the base of your palms over your ears, and apply comfortable pressure in a circular motion.
10. With your thumbs, begin working the area of the bottom of the jaw to the chin. Repeat until this area feels warm or loosened.
11. From your chin, work with your fingertips down the front of your throat to your clavicles—from your shoulders these are the bones resting horizontally across the top of your chest.
12. Grab your right trapezius with your left hand and squeeze. Maintain a firm grip, and turn your head to your left. You should have a firm grip on your trapezius and feel a stretch while your head is turning. Grab the trapezius at different areas close to the neck to the end of the shoulder, and turn your head. Repeat this on the other side.

Your neck should be fairly relaxed now. If not, place a hot pack or hot towel around your neck or head, and repeat any of the steps above to loosen your face, head, neck, and shoulders.

Part Two – Loosening Your Upper Chest, Arms, and Hands

1. Grab your pectoralis major muscle between your thumb and forefinger toward the lateral side. This is just above your armpit.
2. Perform this same technique on the musculature bordering the posterior side of your armpit.

3. Palm your deltoid, and work any tender areas with your thumb. Continue down the arm to the elbow. Again work any tender areas with your thumb or forefinger until the tension is released. You need to work both the inside and outside of the arm.
4. Rotate your forearm so that your inner arm is facing up. Thumb down your inner forearm to the wrist.
5. Rotate your forearm so that the back of your arm is facing you, and palm from the elbow to your wrist. Sitting or kneeling will give you the best leverage for this area.
6. Interlace your fingers and extend your hands out in a motion like cracking your knuckles, but popping your knuckles is not the objective. Work your palm with your thumbs.
7. Grab the fingers of your left hand and grip firmly. "Snap" your fingers by pulling your right hand away quickly. Do this vigorously to release tension in your fingers. Shake your hands when you are finished.
8. If you are kneeling, you can place your arm below your knee and kneel forward onto the forearm. You can do this on the front and back aspects of your forearm. It is best to put your left arm under your right knee and vice versa.

Your upper chest, arms, and hands should be fairly relaxed at this point.

Part Three – Loosening Your Mid-to-Lower Torso, Legs, and Feet

1. Begin working the torso by grabbing your sides with your hands. Gently massage the lateral aspects of your torso from the bottom of the ribs to the hips.
2. Place your thumbs over the area of your kidneys, and gently apply pressure into the area. Now gently rotate your torso in a clockwise rotation nine times; then rotate in the other direction nine times.
3. With the fingers of both hands, begin working the diaphragm, which lies just beneath the ribs. Work from the medial aspect to the lateral aspect.
4. Work the abdominal muscles from the rib cage to your pelvis.
5. From a kneeling position or sitting, begin working the quadriceps with your palms from the hip to the knee. Then thumb down the middle, front, and side of the thigh. You can also work down the leg with your forearm and elbow for deeper pressure.
6. Extend either leg, and work with your palms on both sides of the lower leg. Thumb down the lateral aspect of the leg.
7. Thumb down the front of the feet, working down the line of every toe, and gently pull the toe.
8. Squeeze the back of the thigh to reach the hamstrings. You can interlace your fingers to give you better leverage and deeper pressure. Work the palms of your hands into the hamstrings.
9. To reach the bottom of your foot, you can kneel and reach behind you to thumb down and palm down the bottom of your foot. Crossing your legs will also give you access to the bottom of your feet.
10. Repeat on the other leg.

Your mid-to-lower torso, legs, and feet should be relaxed now.

Part Four – Stretching the Meridians

1.   **Stretching the Lung and Large Intestine Meridians**

Yawning – Induce a yawn by rubbing your face near your nose and mouth. Raise your arms to the side and up. Breathe in through your nose and mouth with your mouth wide open while tilting your head upward and backward. Exhale as you lower your arms.

Bend Over Forward and Raise Your Arms – Stand up. Place your feet shoulder-width apart. Link your thumbs behind you, then exhale and bend forward from your hips, stretching your arms out and up. Your knees can be slightly bent. Breathe, and relax further into it for a few breaths. Uncurl slowly as you exhale.

2.   **Stretching the Stomach and Spleen Meridians**

Leaning Back – From a kneeling position, inhale and on the exhale bring your body forward onto your knees, and stretch your arms back to touch the backs of your heels. You want your hands to be as close to your ankles as possible without pain. Continue this for three breaths, and on an exhale return to a seated position.

Bending Forward – From the kneeling position, with your hands and fingers placed on your abdomen just below your ribcage, exhale as you lean forward at the waist, and apply gentle pressure with your hands into the abdomen. Attempt to touch your head to the floor with this maneuver. When you inhale, stop applying pressure with your hands and lean back.

3.   **Stretching the Bladder and Kidney Meridians**

Sit Down and Touch Your Toes – Sit up as straight as possible. Stretch your legs out to the front; then relax your knees, and let your feet fall outward. Spread your buttocks and ease forward. If this is difficult, sit on the edge of a low cushion. Inhale, and raise your arms straight above your head, palms outward. Then fold forward from your hips, keeping your chest and back extended, and exhaling as you bend. Bring your hands toward your feet, but do not try to grip your legs or pull down. Just stay in the forward bend and breathe. Relax your back, neck, shoulders, arms, and legs. Remain in this position for up to two minutes.

Stand and Rotate From the Hips – Stand with your feet just a little wider than shoulder-width apart. Place your hands over your kidneys, and from this position begin to rotate in both directions from your hips. Keep your chest open and head facing up. This will loosen the lower back and stimulate Chi to the kidneys.

4.   **Stretching the Pericardium and Triple Burner Meridians**

Crossed Legs, Crossed Arms – Sit up straight with legs crossed. Tuck your inside foot in close to the groin. Cross your arms, and hold around your knees. Exhale, and bend forward from the hips. Tuck in your elbows, and relax your upper body, head, and neck. Keep your buttocks on the floor and your pelvis relaxed. Breathe into your *Hara*, the energy center at your navel level. Inhale as you sit up, cross your arms and legs the other way, and repeat.

Swinging Your Arms – Stand with your feet wide apart and parallel. Sink down a little; then relax your pelvis, and tuck in your tailbone. Turn your knees slightly out. Allow your arms to hang at your side, and begin to rotate slowly from the pelvis. Allow your arms to swing naturally.

5. **Stretching the Heart and Small Intestine Meridians**

Advanced Indian Style – Sit with your knees bent and the soles of your feet placed together. If you can't manage this position, sit Indian style. Bring your feet as close to your groin as possible. Let your knees drop. Take in a deep breath, and as you exhale bend forward as far as possible without strain, and let your neck extend. Hold your elbows outside the knees, and breathe in several times in this position. When you are done, inhale and sit up. From this position close your eyes, and pay attention to your breathing. Breathe deeply and steadily for as long as you like, always being aware of your breath.

6. **Stretching the Gall Bladder and Liver Meridians**

Sit and Stretch to the Left and Right – Sit up with your legs stretched out and wide. Turn at the waist to face your left foot. Brace your left hand on the floor behind to lift your trunk and spine. Now wrap your right arm around your chest and ribs, and inhale as you raise your left arm over your head. Exhale slowly, and lower your trunk and left arm in line with your right leg. Rest your left arm over your head, and relax for 2-3 breaths. Come out of this position, and repeat on the other side.

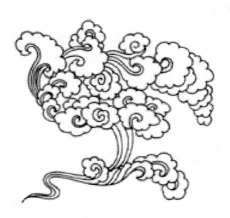

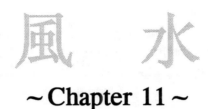

~ Chapter 11 ~

Feng Shui

In the last 25 years acupuncture, acupressure, yoga, martial arts, and Tai Ji have become common along with the concept of yin and yang and the 5 Elements of Traditional Chinese Medicine. In the 1990s the practice of Feng Shui (pronounced fung shway) became popular. Feng Shui is the interaction between you and your environment. It is about creating balance, harmony, and prosperity in your working and living spaces. Feng Shui examines how the energy flow in your environment is affected by the placement of things and objects within it and how these objects interact with and influence your personal energy flow. Whether you are aware of it or not, your environment impacts different areas of your life—health, wealth, family life, relationships, career, and your business.

Feng Shui is a term composed of two Chinese words: Feng (wind) and Shui (water). Wind and water are the two natural elements that flow, move, and circulate everywhere on the planet. They are also the most basic elements required for human survival. The essence of these life-giving elements is, once again, Chi.

Feng Shui and Your Business

Your office—whether an in-home or a commercial space—is a place where your clients can retreat from the pressures of the outside world. It should be a calm, pleasant environment where the Chi flows freely through each room without encountering any harmful obstructions. By learning basic Feng Shui placement and by understanding the *Bagua* map and how to use enhancements and color, you can create balance and harmony in all your living areas, including the space in which you see clients. You can improve energy flow, which will benefit your clients, who come seeking reduced stress and balance in their lives through your help.

Start by Removing Clutter

You need to encourage as much Chi as possible into your office. This enhances your concentration, creativity, and thinking. It also gives you more energy and increases the likelihood of success. It is important to avoid clutter in your office. Clutter constricts Chi and is a source of distraction to you. It creates obstructions in your life. Clear papers and files, as they create clutter that will cause stagnant Chi. Make way for the new by getting rid of the old. Clear out unwanted or broken items, as these only create stagnant energies that may be holding you back. Keep the things that you are attached to in a neat, orderly fashion. When you surround yourself with things that you want and love, your energy will increase every time you see them. Always remove clutter *before* using any Feng Shui enhancements. By doing a major cleaning out you will notice how your life starts to move on.

Space Clearing

Space-clearing techniques are the next tools to use so you can help improve the Chi in your office area. If you are using a portion of your living space to see clients, it is important to clear the space of your energies and that of others who occupy the space with you before your client enters. Negative energy can affect the health and well-being of anyone who enters the room until it is cleared.

There are several ways of clearing space and enhancing Chi for improved health.

1. Orange Peel Cure. Fill a large salad bowl ¾ full of water. Tear the peels off nine oranges and into small pieces, placing them in the bowl. Holding the bowl of water in one hand, dip the fingertips of your other hand into the water. Sprinkle the water around and inside the office, starting at the door until you have circled the entire room and returned to the door. Sprinkle the water everywhere—on the floor, walls, furniture, ceiling, objects, etc.
2. Sound. Circle the room and ring a bell. Hold the thought in your mind of the sound waves carrying your intention of clearing the space throughout every part of the area. End by moving the bell in a figure eight, which completes the clearing and "ties the room off."
3. Smudging. Light sage, and as it smolders walk around the circumference of the room, waving it in all the corners.
4. Essential Oil. Spray a room, using a water mister and a few drops of essential oil. For healing, use lavender essential oil. After an illness spray with eucalyptus, lemon, or rosemary. To increase life energy use orange, lemongrass, lime, or peppermint.

With all of these cures, end by vocally blessing your space with a prayer, affirmation, chant, or other spiritual tradition. Visualize, and feel that the blessing has been completely successful and your space cleansed.

Bagua Map

The *Bagua* Map is a visual tool that you can apply to any space—your entire home, office building, a lot, or just a room. It can be either a square-, rectangle-, or octagon-shaped tool. It is placed over any space and divides it into nine areas that correspond to nine areas in your life. This helps you pinpoint areas that need change. For example, suppose you need more money. First you would find the area that is related to wealth, assess the current energy conditions, and then make changes to enhance the energy in that area. The meaning of the squares are slightly different for business than they are for your personal living space.

To use the *Bagua* Map:

1. Always place the map in relation to the main, or most used, entrance to the room. This is where the main flow of energy enters.
2. If the room is not square or rectangular in shape, square it off. To square off your office, draw lines off the corners to complete the rectangle.
3. Divide the area into 9 equal squares.
4. Overlay the *Bagua* life areas in the squares with the bottom of the map aligned with the front door or the entrance most often used.
5. Look for any missing areas. For instance, if your office is L-shaped, one or more life areas are missing, which could negatively impact your business. Missing areas in your office can reflect missing energy in the life area affected.
6. Choose the areas you wish to focus on for improvement.
7. Choose Feng Shui cures to balance, enhance, or help the Chi to flow better.
8. End by visualizing your desired goal and vocally blessing the change, or write it out in the form of an affirmation.

Ten Feng Shui Cures For Your Office

Feng Shui cures or enhancements can involve:

1. *Location:*
   Within the home, an office that is close to the front of the house nearest the street and outside world is best. This will also keep the office energies separate from the rest of the house. Think outside the box. A living room doesn't have to be a living room. Perhaps one of the bedrooms or dining room could work better for an in-home office. To encourage the success of your business, your in-home office is best located in the Wealth, Fame, or Career areas of the *Bagua* map, but if it isn't, enhance those areas within your office space.
2. *Plants:*
   Attract vital energy with healthy-looking plants—real or silk—avoiding dried plants as they are dead and do not promote Chi. Pictures of flowers can also be used when correct lighting is a problem. A jade plant—which symbolizes wealth—is excellent for the office area.
3. *Color:*
   The colors associated with the 5 Elements and a particular life area can be used to enhance Chi. Color can be applied to the walls, through art, rugs, in a candle, or used as a decorating accent in pillows or towels, etc.
4. *Mirrors:*
   If when sitting at your desk you sit with your back to the door, on the wall you face, install a mirror that reflects the door.
5. *Crystals:*
   A faceted crystal ball hanging from the ceiling can help energize an entire room. The energy of crystals can stimulate wealth and success. Hanging a crystal in the Career sector of your house also attracts Chi and provides extra energy to help you in your work.
6. *5 Elements:*
   Placing a representation of the 5 Elements in a particular *Bagua* square will enhance that area. For instance, placing something with wood—a sculpture, picture frame, piece of wooden

furniture, etc., will enhance the career area. Placing a metal box containing a few coins in the wealth corner of your desk activates your work area.

7. *Water:*

Water signifies wealth, and flowing water creates your cash flow. Place a water element, either a table fountain or picture of moving water, near your front door and/or in your office. Fountains that circulate water into a pool symbolize the accumulation of money. The water should flow toward you to bring an abundant flow of money and prosperity. Also, in a bathroom keep the toilet seat down and the door shut when not in use to minimize the amount of positive energy being flushed away.

8. *Wind chimes:*

Metal wind chimes are also good in the wealth corner or as you enter your home. The sound reinforces your intent to attract wealth. Another use of sound is to place your phone in the wealth area of your desk to enhance your business.

9. *Light:*

Make sure your front door, the career, and the wealth areas in your *Bagua* map are well lit to encourage Chi. Use candles in the colors of the 5 elements of red, green, yellow, white, and black to attract Chi. If the wealth and prosperity area is dark, use a low-wattage bulb in a lamp in that area and keep it on all the time to enhance the flow of Chi.

10. *Words:*

Have quotes, affirmations, and sayings pertaining to career, success, and wealth around you to focus your thoughts, consciously or unconsciously, on the enhancement of these qualities.

Commanding Position: The heart of your workplace

In your office, the most important item is the position of your desk. Good positioning of your desk can make the difference between an easy, smooth, and growing career or one filled with hardships, setbacks, and problems.

Your desk should be:

1. Positioned to see the office door and allow you to see as much of the room as possible. If the door is to your back, install a mirror on the wall you face that reflects the door.
2. As far as possible from the door, but not be in the direct path of the door, nor against a wall so that you cannot approach it from both sides.
3. Solid and big enough for your work. Buy the best wood desk you can afford.
4. Placed in either the career or wealth areas of the *Bagua* of the room or the home if possible.

These same rules apply when you are working on clients whether they are on a table or sitting in a chair. You should be able to see the door and have a wall behind you for support. Also watch out for sharp edges on tables and desks, or walls. These angles are known as "poison arrows" and send negative Chi your way. Re-position furniture to avoid them, or soften the angles by placing a large plant in front of them.

Feng Shui & Health

Chi works on many different levels and affects everything in and around us. It affects our emotions, our physical strength, even our resistance to disease. A contributing factor to health and well-being is strong internal Chi reinforced by an environment that has good Feng Shui. A beneficial concentration of Chi can help encourage the body's natural healing process. Implementing good Feng Shui changes, coupled with focused intentions, can strengthen the Chi in our environment and help to balance out our lives. One of Feng Shui's main points is that nothing exists outside you that does not already exist inside you.

Health is dependent on every aspect of life working well. The environment of our homes is significant to our health, but when we are sick it becomes even more important because our home is usually the place where we go to rest and recuperate. It is difficult to heal in an environment that is devoid of life force and does not support us physically, emotionally, and spiritually. When we are ill, our Chi is compromised and low. It is at this time that we are in need of additional life force from our environment to aid in the healing process. During both the awake and sleep states the body will seek to gain energy and life force from its surroundings. This is why it is especially important to assess and then enhance life force elements inside the room in which you sleep.

When we view the *Bagua* map of the home, we see it is recommended that the Family and Health *gua* be activated by healthy, thriving plants—because plants are symbolic of health, growth, and wood, the element which governs this area. The best indoor plants are those with rounded leaves. If you use cut flowers to enhance this area, make sure they are always fresh, as dead flowers deplete Chi.

There are many levels in which Feng Shui can be applied to health by placing the *Bagua* map over your home and/or office environment and then using the additional information associated with the various *guas* for the different levels of our being—the mental, emotional, and spiritual components.

Five Levels of Feng Shui Applications:

1st Level—your physical environment (home and/or office)

- Any missing *Bagua* areas in your environment due to physical layout—either in home, apartment, or office—can reflect areas of the body where Chi is also missing.
- Clutter, and where it is found in your home or office, means stagnation in a part of your life and body.

2nd Level—your physical body

- The 9 *guas* are each associated with a body part.
- The 9 *guas* are associated with the 5 Elements of TCM, which in turn is linked to meridians that are associated with specific organs.

3rd Level—your emotional and mental states

- Chi affects your emotions and attitude about life. Each *gua* can be linked to psychological issues.
- Depression is associated with stagnant Chi, robbing you of power to live life fully. Life seems dull and appears to conspire against you. When your internal Chi is strong, you enjoy challenge, facing life with courage, and the ability to act.

4th Level—energetically linked to your spiritual sense and well-being

- The chakras of Indian Ayurvedic medicine interact with the Feng Shui of your environment, and together they energetically create your life. Chakras are energy centers whose location in the body often correlates with the organs. Chakras can also be linked to the *guas*.
- The *guas* are associated with the 5 Elements of TCM.

5th Level—color is another form of life force or energy

- Color is another important component in how completely and quickly you heal.
- The *guas* are associated with the colors of the chakras and 5 Elements.

Intentions

Intentions are very important because energy follows thought. Intentions are used to accompany any Feng Shui enhancement—whether for environment or health. Focus your attention on intention. Energy supports our intention. Visualization, guided imagery, and affirmations can also be used as ways of focusing intention.

As you do a health enhancement, focus your intentions by:

1. Visualizing the organ or body area that is ill in a healthy state or moving toward health;
2. Feeling your Chi becoming stronger;
3. Seeing yourself once again doing things that you were able to do before you became ill;
4. Seeing yourself fully recovered, enjoying life; and
5. Expressing gratitude for your renewing health.

Practical Use:

When we find an area of sensitivity while doing bodywork, by consulting the *Bagua* map where the organ or body part is located, we can link that sensitivity to a living space to see if there is stagnant Chi in a corresponding area or if the area is missing from the floor plan. Or, using TCM, by finding the meridian or organ that is unbalanced we can look at the *Bagua* map and find in what *gua* it is located and then see if the client is experiencing physical, mental, or emotional problems associated with that area. Either way, enhancements can be selected to strengthen the Chi in the living area, which in turn may promote all levels of the human being toward health.

Feng Shui offers a way of beginning to unravel the mystery of illness. This way of working, however, is not to be taken as a "cookie cutter" approach. If something is out of balance, we must consider the entire person, not just where the imbalance is found. Also, remember, if something is unbalanced in one area, this will cause something else to be unbalanced to compensate. Think in terms of the relationships found in TCM. Combining bodywork with Feng Shui enlarges the view we hold of our clients. When using Feng Shui on ourselves or others, always work holistically. Feng Shui may not be the whole story, but it is well worth exploring for contributing factors when there is disease present.

Feng Shui is a life study. It is a multifaceted tool that enables you to understand how your environment affects you and how to rearrange your life to a new higher level. Feng Shui leads you to new discoveries and knowledge, and gives you tools to enhance your life and business. With many of the Feng Shui cures costing little or nothing, you probably will find you have lots of things to use as cures already, just in the wrong places. We have literally only scratched the surface here. For more information you can read books, watch videos, or engage a professional Feng Shui consultant. Feng Shui is a valuable asset for your business, life, and health.

BUSINESS BAGUA MAP
© Issel 2003

Wealth/ Prosperity/ Abundance	Fame/ Reputation/ Luck/ Integrity/ Future	Partnerships/ Relationships
Cash flow/ financial status/ raising money for a special purpose or project	Marketing/ public relations/ word-of-mouth advertising/ market position	The relationship between business partners/ the relationship between business owners and their clients
Colors: Blues/ Purples/ Reds	Reds	Reds/ Pinks/ Whites
5 Elements: Wood/Fire	Fire	Fire/Metal
Family	Health	Creativity/ Communications
Employees/ management/ vendors/ co-workers/ those with whom you share office space	Your physical health on all levels: physical, mental, emotional, spiritual	To enhance creativity in yourself and others/ to enhance communications/ to move more quickly in business, with more fluidity
Colors: Blues/ Greens	Yellows/ Earth tones	Whites/ Pastels
5 Elements: Wood	Earth	Metal
Knowledge	Career	Helpful People/ Travel/ New Directions
Flow of information/ business data/ computer networks/ Internet/ education/ wisdom	Relationship with the world outside/ your life's journey/ business success	Networking/ colleagues/ business associates/ mentors/ clients
Colors: Blacks/ Blues/ Greens	Blacks/ Navy/ Dark tones	Whites/ Grays/ Blacks
5 Elements: Wood/Water	Water	Water/Metal

Align the main door, entering the room along this line.

HEALTH BAGUA MAP

© Issel 2003

Gua	Wealth/ Prosperity/ Abundance	Fame/ Reputation/ Luck/ Integrity/ Future	Partnerships/ Relationships
Psychology:	Survival	Mental illness	Mother/ relationships
Anatomy:	Hips/ pelvis/ bones	Eyes	Stomach/ organs
Disorders of:	Genitals/ rectum/ blood disorders/ birth/ pelvic cavity	CNS & circulatory systems/ cranial cavity/ blood disorders/ immune system	Mid-back/ organs in abdominal cavity
Chakra: Location: Color:	1st – Root Chakra Base of spine Red	7th – Crown Chakra Top of head Purple	4th – Heart Chakra Center of chest Green
Feng Shui colors: 5 Elements:	Blues/ Purples/ Reds Wood/Fire	Reds Fire	Reds/ Pinks/ Whites Fire/Metal
Gua	Family	Health	Creativity/ Children/ Communications
Psychology:	Social center/ family/ past/ depression		Future
Anatomy:	Feet		Mouth
Disorders of:	Reproductive organs/ spleen/ large intestine/ kidneys/ urinary tract/ lower back/ appendix	Overall health and vitality	Neck/ teeth/ gums/ jaw/ thyroid/ parathyroid/ hypothalamus
Chakra: Location: Color:	2nd – Sacrum Chakra Below navel Orange	Golden Light	5th – Throat Chakra Throat Sky Blue
Feng Shui colors: 5 Elements:	Blues/ Greens Wood	Yellows/ Earth tones Earth	Whites/ Pastels Metal
Gua	Knowledge/ Spirituality	Career	Helpful People/ Travel/ New Directions
Psychology:		Anxiety	Father
Anatomy:	Hands	Ears	Head
Disorders of:	Hands/ wrists/ arms/ neurological & sense systems/ forehead/ nose	Adrenals/ stomach/ liver/ pancreas/ gall bladder/ mid-back/ small intestines/ ears	Central nervous system/ systemic illness/ top of head
Chakra: Location: Color:	6th – Third Eye Between eyebrows Indigo	3rd – Will center Solar plexus Yellow	8th – Transpersonal center 6" above head White light
Feng Shui colors: 5 Elements:	Blacks/ Blues/ Greens Wood/Water	Blacks/ Navy/ Dark tones Water	Whites/ Grays/ Blacks Water/Metal

Place front door or entrance to a room along this line.

Bibliography

Beinfield, Harriet with Korngold, Efrem. *Between Heaven and Earth*. New York: Ballantine Books, 1991.

Biofeld, John. *Taoism: The Road to Immortality*. Boulder: Shamnala Publications, 1980.

Chang Chung-yuan. *Creativity and Taoism*. New York: The Julian Press, 1963.

Chu Hsi. The Great Extreme (or First Cause of Existence). *The Shrine of Wisdom* 10, 1929.

Collins, Terah Kathryn. *The Western Guide to Feng Shui*. Hay House, 1996.

Collins, Terah Kathryn. *The Western Guide to Feng Shui Room by Room*. Hay House, 1999.

Collins, Terah Kathryn. *The Western Guide to Feng Shui For Prosperity*. Hay House, 2002.

Dubitsky, Carl. *Bodywork Shiatsu*. Rochester: Healing Arts Press, 1977. (meridian drawings adapted from pgs.46 – 55)

Dunn, David. *Qi-Gong: An Introduction to the Science of Self-cultivation* (unpublished article).

Exkert, Achim. *Chinese Medicine for Beginners*. Prima Publishing, 1996.

Gach, Michael Reed. *Acupressure's Potent Points*. Bantam Books, 1990.

Gach, Michael Reed. *Intermediate & Advanced Acupressure Course Booklet*. Michael Reed Gach, 1984.

Gerber, Richard. *Vibrational Medicine*. Santa Fe: Bear & Company, 1996.

Hsu, Hong-Yen with Preacher, William. *Chen's History of Chinese Medical Science*. Modern Drug Publishers Co., 1977.

Huai Nan Tsze. The History of Great Light. *The Shrine of Wisdom* 18, 1937.

Issel, Christine. Feng Shui Health & Business Maps. *Reflexology Today*. Winter 2002 & Summer 2003. ARCB. Arvada, CO, 2003

Issel, Christine & Rodgers, Sandra. *Reflexognosy: A Shift in Paradigm*. Sacramento: New Frontier Publishing, 2000

Kaptchik, Ted J. *The Web That Has No Weaver—Understanding Chinese Medicine*. New York: Congdon & Weed, Inc., 1983. (partial *Zang Fu* information adapted from pgs. 54 – 69)

Bibliography (continued)

Kennedy, David Daniel. *Feng Shui for Dummies*. New York: Hungry Minds, 2001.

Ko-Hsuan. The Classic of Purity. *The Shrine of Wisdom* 11, 1930.

Lundberg, Paul. *The Book of Shiatsu*. London: Gaia Books Limited, 1992.

Maciocia, Giovanni. *The Foundations of Chinese Medicine*. Edinburgh: Churchill Livingstone, 1989. (partial *Zang Fu* information adapted from pgs. 67 – 125)

Masunaga, Shizuto with Ohashi, Wataru. *Zen Shiatsu*. Japan Publications, 1977.

Merton, Thomas (translator). *The Way of Chuang Tzu*. New York: New Directions Books, 1969.

Rosbach, Sarah. *Interior Design with Feng Shui*. New York: Penguin Putnam, 2000.

SantoPietro, Nancy. *Feng Shui and Health*. New York: Three Rivers Press, 2002. (Health Bagua Map adapted from pgs. 216-217, 233)

Teeguarden, Ron. *Chinese Tonic Herbs*. Japan Publications, Inc., 1994. (Taoist cosmology adapted from pgs. 21 – 33)

Webster, Richard. *Feng Shui for the Workplace*. St. Paul, MN: Llewellyn Publications, 1998.

Xinnong, Cheng. *Chinese Acupressure and Moxibustion*. Foreign Language Press, 1987.

Yang, Jwing-Ming. *Chinese Qigong Massage*. YMAA Publishing Center, 1992.

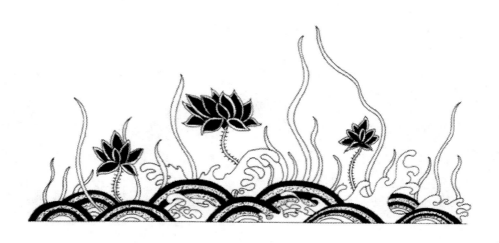

Special Notes

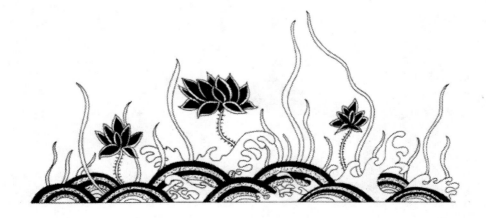

Special Notes

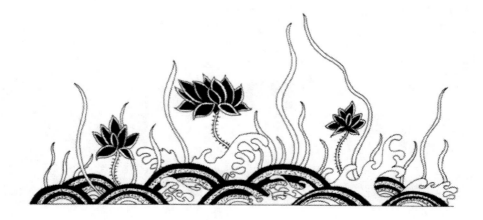

Special Notes

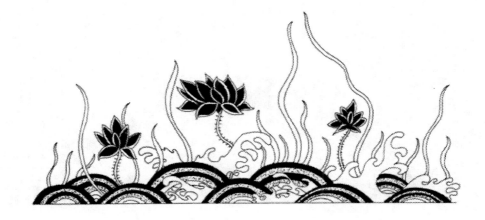

Special Notes

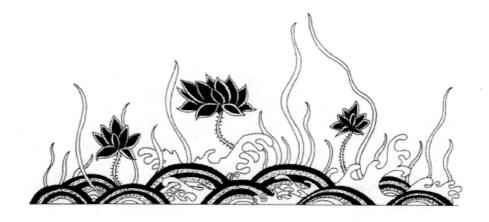